D1190899

"A superb self-efficacy tool for anyone who has a chronic illness. Fennell's four-phase approach adds the dimension of dealing with the social milieu in which the chronically ill person must function."

—Miryam Ehrlich Williamson, author, *Fibromyalgia: A Comprehensive Approach* and *The Fibromyalgia Relief Book*

"Pat Fennell has succinctly addressed the problems faced by people with chronic illnesses and their providers. . . . The Phase Model ties it all together! I will recommend it to colleagues and friends. A great tool in our treatment toolkit and an excellent aid to any patient who has a chronic illness."

—Donald Uslan, M.A., M.B.A., Medical Psychotherapist and Rehabilitation Counselor Northwest Counseling Associates

The Chronic Illness Workbook

Strategies and Solutions for Taking Back Your Life

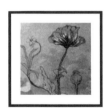

PATRICIA A. FENNELL, MSW, CSW-R

NEW HARBINGER PUBLICATIONS, INC.

Publisher's Note

This publication is designed to provide accurate and authoritative information in regard to the subject matter covered. It is sold with the understanding that the publisher is not engaged in rendering psychological, financial, legal, or other professional services. If expert assistance or counseling is needed, the services of a competent professional should be sought.

Distributed in the U.S.A. by Publishers Group West; in Canada by Raincoast Books; in Great Britain by Airlift Book Company, Ltd.; in South Africa by Real Books, Ltd.; in Australia by Boobook; and in New Zealand by Tandem Press.

Copyright © 2001 by Patricia A. Fennell
New Harbinger Publications, Inc.
5674 Shattuck Avenue
Oakland, CA 94609

Cover design by Salmon Studios
Text design by Tracy Marie Powell

Library of Congress Card Catalog Number: 00-132291
ISBN 1-57224-264-7 Paperback

03   02   01
10   9   8   7   6   5   4   3   2   1
First printing

*My barn having burned to the ground
I can now see the moon.*

—Anonymous

To my patients and mentors
who are often one and the same

Contents

PART III

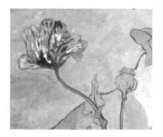

I want to thank my irreplaceable teachers and guides, starting more or less from the beginning: Dorothy, Nora, Anna, Megen, Sister Francis Eustace, Helena, and of course Pearl.

I also want to thank my invaluable supporters and truly stalwart friends: Kathy Sarafino, Judy, Dr. Carolyn Grosvenor, and Dr. Leonard Buchakjian; Wally, Kathy, Leslie, John, and Margaret; my sisters Cindy and Paula, and my abiding Erick.

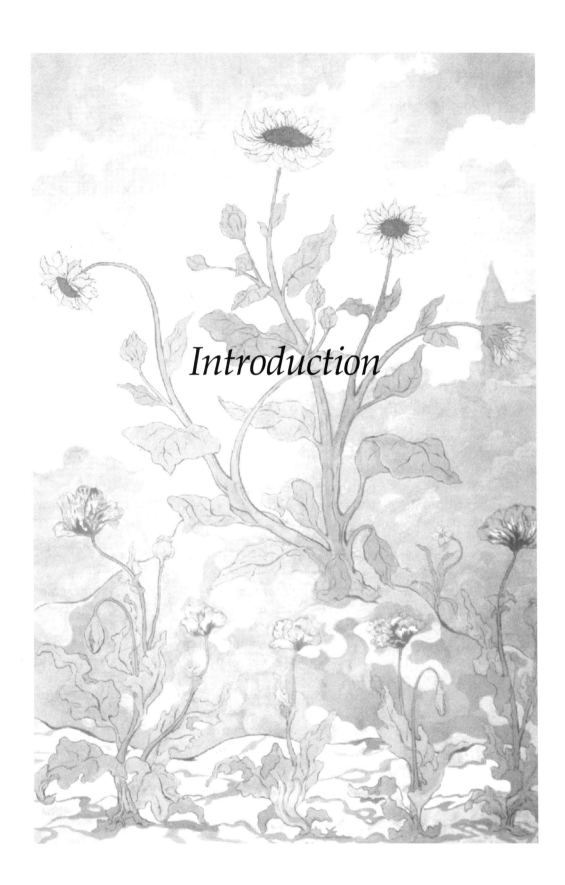

Introduction

Voices of Chronic Illness

Trauma of Onset: Paula

"It was as if my world turned upside down and inside out," Paula said. "When I awoke that morning, the room was changed, my mind was different, I wasn't thinking right, I couldn't find words. My body was filled with pain, and it was racing and burning. I couldn't move my limbs right—they wouldn't obey me. It was like every part of me was foreign. I didn't know how to understand it."

Perhaps this is how chronic illness began for you—out of the blue, totally debilitating, and emotionally devastating. Here was Paula, an articulate, intelligent, capable woman, telling me about the onset of her illness six years earlier. I watched her fill with fear, even terror, simply in the telling. The nightmare might have occurred yesterday, she was so frightened at the prospect of such things ever happening again. She still felt this way even though she'd come to a place where her life was beginning, once again, to be fulfilling.

Loss of Old Self: Joan

"I was talking on the phone with Cindy," Joan said, "and she was telling me about the new man in her life and about how they were trying to blend their work styles and homes and furniture and all. Then she asked me about my life. I didn't know what to say. Finally I said that I didn't really want to lay all my symptoms on her. But as a matter of fact, I was thinking about how I had to choose between washing my hair or going to the store. I didn't have the energy to do both. Still, I'd been able to do a little picking up, and I thought that showed progress. She interrupted me and what she said—I can't remember the exact words now—shocked me. She said, 'It's like the Joan I knew is dead. I don't recognize you anymore. It's like you're a completely different person.'"

If you have a chronic illness, you may have suffered this kind of wounding yourself. Joan was already suffering from her illness and from her personal experience of losing the self that she used to be. Now, in addition, she was hurt by the insensitivity of her friend. And even though Cindy had suffered a loss, too (losing the person she had known Joan to be), it's unfortunate that she wasn't capable of extending her former affection to the person Joan had been forced by her illness to become. Perhaps, like Joan, you also recognize that your illness has changed you, that you're not the person you used to be, much as you'd like to be. But things don't need to stop there. It's possible for people with chronic illnesses to understand their condition so clearly that their lives not only become manageable but are truly meaningful again as well.

Stigmatized at Work: Sarah

"The word finally got around at work," Sarah said, "that the reason I'd missed so much work was because I had chronic fatigue syndrome. And then I began to notice that the girl I shared an office with was staying as far away from me as possible. She seemed really upset when I used one of the mugs that we all use for coffee. I joked with her that she was acting like I had the plague. She got really flustered but kind of mad, too. She said she'd read an article that said my problem was contagious, and she didn't want to get it. Nothing I said made any difference."

You're probably aware that TV shows and the tabloid press often dramatize degrading, demeaning, and mistaken notions about chronic illnesses. These stories feed people's fears and anxieties. In the profit-driven atmosphere of the entertainment industry, sensationalism pays better than truth, even if some people suffer as a result. The stigma associated with many chronic illnesses causes a lot of people to try to hide their condition or to feel enormous shame about it. But there's no reason for anyone to accept prejudice in any form. You can learn to protect your rights and stand up for your emotional well-being, too.

Rejected by Loved Ones: Jill

Jill's partner Robert said, "You know, this isn't the life I signed up for. This isn't the woman I married. This isn't what I expected. I want my old life back. I want my old wife back. She used to make lunch occasionally. We used to be able to make love. We used to be able to go out. Now everything is a struggle, everything has to be planned ahead of time, thought through. It's tiresome, it's aggravating."

Family members also suffer when you have a chronic illness. With guidance and help, many learn to deal with the new realities and sustain their affections. If they can't, you need to learn how to maintain your self-esteem and recognize that you can find companions who will love the person you are now.

Disbelieved by Doctors: Karen

"I can't believe it," Karen said. "The health-care workers had never seen me in my wheelchair before, and I think it freaked them out. When I came into the waiting room, they all came rushing up to me, asking me how I was. Well, the truth is that I was embarrassed. I don't like to use the wheelchair, so I only use it when I'm really having trouble walking. I hate how people respond to it, because it reminds me of how unstable I really am. So when they all started saying stuff about it, it made tears come to my eyes. When I went in for my exam, the doctor said I was obviously depressed and insisted that I take Prozac to help with my 'symptoms.' God, you know you get tears in your eyes for a real good reason, and they want to medicate you. I can't believe it. She gave me Prozac!"

As you probably know very well, not all doctors and nurses behave intelligently or sympathetically with the chronically ill. It is therefore extremely important for you to find health-care professionals who understand chronic illness in all its dimensions. Many clinicians are more than willing to learn. This book includes information for you to share with them that will help you work together as an effective team.

Never Got a Life: Ken

"I've been in this room, pretty much in bed, for a few years," Ken, who is seventeen, said. "I use my computer to talk to people, friends I used to have at school and people I met through the chat rooms who have the same kind of illness. I also write letters to people. But I really haven't been to school in years, and I miss it. I try to keep my spirits up by going on the computer and writing every day, but it gets hard sometimes. I wonder what other kids are doing. Now they are getting ready to go to college and I'm not. I worry about being left behind and where I'm going to go."

Some young people who are chronically ill never get the chance to develop an ordinary life in the first place. Yet even if you are young, or the person you care for is, you can also navigate the phases of the illness to arrive at a life worth living.

Core Realities of Chronic Illness

You've probably recognized yourself or someone you love in these stories. Each one illustrates events that are commonplace for the chronically ill and the people who love them. Gradually, over years of listening, I found that certain core realities about chronic illness began to emerge out of all the experiences I was hearing. And I found that when chronically ill people are helped to deal with these and other issues, they can move forward with a positive spirit into enriching lives, despite their sometimes significant disabilities.

What are the core realities involved in living with a chronic illness?

Onset

As your illness begins, it can cause you growing fear and suffering. This includes physical pain, changes in your ability to think, mood swings, physical limitations and enormous frustration, denial, and grief. Your illness may come on suddenly or gradually. But when you finally acknowledge that something is truly wrong with you, the moment of recognition itself also hurts you. It can cause a trauma, a shock. It can be likened to a physical and emotional earthquake.

Rejection

In addition, just about everyone who is chronically ill suffers some form of rejection by other people, especially people they care about. This rejection can come about for any number of reasons. Perhaps your partner, like Robert in Jill's story above, can't stand the change that illness brings to your relationship. Perhaps, like Robert eventually did, your partner leaves you, blaming you for destroying the life the two of you shared. While people like Robert may seem selfish and unwilling to do any emotional heavy lifting, it's also true that Robert did lose the life he was living and the partner he had married.

Loss of Self

Perhaps, like Joan, you've lost old friends, people who can't stretch their affection to love the you that you've become. Actually Joan was just as confused as Cindy about how to remain friends because Joan knew she wasn't herself anymore. She wasn't feeling or thinking or acting like she used to. But it took Cindy's stark words to make Joan really understand this core reality about chronic illness. Once you have a chronic illness, you lose your former self, the person you used to be before the illness. You can't do many of the things you used to do. It seems like you have to give up all your former plans for the future.

Role Changes

Your condition may drastically change how well you can fulfill your roles—as partner, worker, friend, parent, neighbor. Maybe now you can't make love, or at least not the way you used to. Maybe you can't do your old job anymore, and you worry about how you'll manage without that income. Maybe you're too exhausted nowadays to go to the movies or dinner with your friends. Maybe you can't get to teacher conferences at school anymore. Maybe, like Sarah, some co-workers or neighbors steer clear of you now because your condition scares them or perhaps just embarrasses them.

Identity Confusion

Even if the changes in your life aren't that severe—your partner doesn't divorce you; you are able to continue working, if only part-time—the person you used to be is gone. This can cause you enormous grief and great worry. If you aren't who you used to be, who are you? Who will you become? What kind of life can you possibly have, given your illness, given your restrictions?

Cultural Stigmatization

Maybe you've got co-workers, neighbors, or friends who avoid you or think less of you because they believe misinformation they've read in the supermarket tabloids or hear on TV. Sometimes doctors and other health-care professionals disbelieve or disparage conditions that are unfamiliar to them. Even if they are sympathetic, they may treat your problem as something "in your mind," something emotional or caused by stress. Some chronic illnesses have only recently been identified as medical conditions. It can take decades for society and the culture at large to accept a new disease as something "real," deserving of sympathy and understanding. If you have a chronic illness, the shame it may cause you can be one of the most painful aspects of your condition.

No "Normal" Development

Perhaps, like Ken, you've been ill since childhood. Ken never had the chance to develop a so-called "normal" life, to grow into manhood, to develop an ordinary identity. Children, teenagers, young adults with chronic illnesses have to wrestle with somewhat different questions. What is "normal"? Will you ever be able to go to school? Will you ever complete school? Will you ever have a girlfriend or boyfriend? And at the same time that you're trying to answer these questions, you're wrestling with tremendous loneliness, loss, envy, and anger because you've been deprived of so much.

Disbelief and Suspicion

You've probably had experiences with people disbelieving your symptoms, like Karen did. This experience sheds light on yet another core reality of chronic illness. Some people—health-care providers, trusted family members, friends—will misunderstand you, not believe you, and stigmatize you. Primarily this occurs because of ignorance. But even when they should know better, some people will regard you as crazy or malingering. Some people will question whether you're really ill, and some will just regard you with suspicion.

Clinically Induced Trauma

Karen regularly told her doctor and the doctor's staff that there were days when she couldn't walk at all. Yet it was only when she appeared in a wheelchair, making a strong visual impact on these health-care professionals, that they finally believed she did have difficulty walking. Only then did they show concern and begin asking her questions. Karen was annoyed that they either hadn't listened to what she'd told them over and over again, or else they hadn't believed her. An even bigger blow came when the doctor ordered her to take Prozac. Karen felt that she ought to be allowed to cry sometimes, that she had good reasons to cry. Instead, she came away from the office with the distinct message from her doctor that her tears were a sign of behavior that had to be medicated away. Most health-care professionals are decent, well-trained individuals. Yet in this instance, quite unintentionally, they hurt Karen seriously. It was more than just a wasted visit for her and likely a source of frustration for her health-care providers, too. Karen and her husband now feel that they've got to prepare themselves emotionally before every health-care visit. As a consequence, they're reluctant to go at all, even though Karen requires medical monitoring and treatment.

Transforming Your Illness Experience

To sum up, if you are chronically ill, you can experience shock and trauma at the onset of your disease. You may also experience the rejection of others and the loss of yourself and the life you've known until now. You're almost inevitably going to experience some disbelief, bias, and outright stigmatization from those you love, depend on, work with, and sometimes receive care from, such as your doctor or therapist. If you've been sick through your childhood, teen, or young-adult years, you've also suffered from never having had the chance to make an ordinary life at all. And, finally, your chronic illness has a severe impact and creates loss for those around you—your family members, your friends, your co-workers, your boss, and your health-care providers.

But this doesn't have to be the whole story. You can help make your life better. By taking the different approach offered in this book, you can reduce your fear and pain, recreate a new self, and arrive at a life that gives you satisfaction and purpose.

The Four-Phase Approach

The four-phase approach presented this book gives you a way to rewrite the story of you and your illness. At the end of your narrative, you'll be able to care about yourself and to live a meaningful, fulfilling life in safety and dignity. The four-phase method helps you move away from the shame, even self-loathing, that so often accompanies chronic illness. By following its strong, positive models and clear, sensible advice on how to deal with practical problems, this book can help you escape from the exhausting effort of trying to pretend that you can still do everything you always used to—what's called trying to "pass." Instead you'll construct a new life that takes into consideration the realities of your illness and its cycles of relapse and recovery. In the process of building a sustainable life, you also create new meaning for your existence. Once again you'll see yourself in a positive way. Ultimately, you'll be able to integrate your illness experience into a complete and full new life. Even though your illness may take up a large part of your time and attention, it will not define your existence. It will simply be one of many aspects of your new self.

How This Book Will Help You

Society doesn't prepare anyone to cope with chronic illness. You didn't get any information about it in high school or college health classes. Even the people who currently provide care for the chronically ill receive little training in the real experience of chronic illness. And this is true even though doctors are diagnosing chronic illness at a sharply increasing rate. In fact, the *Journal of the American Medical Association* recently stated that nearly half of the population of the United States suffers from some form of chronic illness.[1]

As one of the millions of Americans who suffers from chronic illness, you know that it can be a traumatizing, life-changing experience. Yet it seems that there are few tools to help you and your family deal with these new realities. Society appears to have only two approaches to illness: either people get better, with or without a doctor's help, or they die.

If you have a chronic illness, you don't fit either pattern. Instead you go through cycles of relapse and recovery. As the old joke says, "The good news is that you're not going to die—and the bad news is that you're not going to die."

This book gives you a positive, realistic alternative to your existing cultural choices. It defines four phases of change that can occur in everyone with a chronic illness. As you navigate through them, you create a narrative or story in which you proudly define your new self and your new life. For each phase the book describes what you can expect from yourself, and from those immediately around you, in your workplace and from the society at large. The book also gives you detailed methods to use for working successfully with your health-care providers.

By reading this book and taking the recommended steps, you'll be able to:

- Recognize the important physical and social differences between acute illness and chronic illness

- Recognize the basic realities of chronic illness, including trauma and cultural stigmatization

---

1 Hoffman, C., D. Rice, and Sung Hy. 1997. Persons with chronic conditions: Their prevalence and costs. *Journal of the American Medical Association* 277(3):375–376.

- Improve your day-to-day life as you cope with your chronic illness

- Learn specific strategies, skills, and coping tools for each phase of the chronic illness

- Involve your family and friends effectively so that they can help you progress through each phase of the four-phase process

- Develop an appropriate and more effective relationship with your health-care providers

- Integrate your illness experience into a meaningful new life rather than hopelessly pursue an unattainable cure

How This Book Is Organized

Part I covers two important topics. Chapter 1 helps you understand what it means to be chronically ill and to treat chronic illness in the health-care system today. It also teaches you how attitudes and beliefs shape the chronic illness experience. Chapter 2 helps you understand chronic illness from the four-phase perspective.

Part II describes the four phases in greater detail. There are exercises in each phase that will help you to accomplish the tasks that will help you move forward into the next phase. I suggest that you make several copies of each blank exercise. You will want to fill in some of them several times. Chapter 3 discusses phase one, "The Crisis Phase." Here you move from the onset of the illness to an emergency state where your task and that of the people around you is to cope with this trauma. Chapter 4 presents phase two, "The Stabilization Phase." In this phase you learn how to make order out of chaos. You begin stabilizing your situation and creating a new life. Chapter 5 covers phase three, "The Resolution Phase." Here you start to make meaning out of your suffering, and you begin to comprehend how the illness fits into the new life you're forging. Chapter 6 brings you to phase four, "The Integration Phase," in which you learn how to integrate the life you had before your illness with the new life that you have now.

Part III covers a number of special topics. Chapter 7, "Getting Help and How to Manage It," guides you through the health-care system. It helps you identify what kind of assistance you need, whom to get it from, and how to get it. You'll learn when to obtain additional opinions and when to change doctors. Other topics include an introduction to health-care relationship etiquette and alternative medical care. Chapter 8, "Couples, Caregivers, and Kids," discusses the relationship between partners when one is chronically ill. It considers the role of caregiver, noting especially the role of caring for a child who is chronically ill. The chapter includes such issues as sexuality, how you as caregiver must care for yourself, and how to establish boundaries and set limits. It considers loss, grief, adjustment, how to respond to the needs of your healthy children, the extended family, concerns about schooling, and negotiating developmental milestones. Chapter 9, "Chronic Illness and Special Situations," gives you or the chronically ill person you care for pointers on how to deal with major life changes like getting married, retiring, moving, and also with matters like traveling, dining out with friends, and occasions like graduations, weddings, and funerals. It also deals with matters like attending school or handling your job. Chapter 10, "Countertransference and Health-Care Professionals," will help you and your health-care providers develop an appropriate, effective working relationship. Read this chapter carefully and then discuss it with your health-care professionals. It will help you work together as a team.

The four-phase method shows you how to rewrite your personal chronic illness story and guides you along your individual chronic-illness journey. As the unknown becomes more comprehensible, you'll experience less fear and anxiety. As you locate your personal narrative in the evolving process of the four phases, you'll see order and meaning emerging out of your sometimes traumatic experiences. Working through the exercises included in the chapters will help diminish your confusion, and you'll find your experiences have greater coherence.

It's my hope that this book will give you a way to validate the realities of your experiences, stabilize and structure your life, develop meaning for your experiences, and ultimately enjoy the whole, complete life that you deserve.

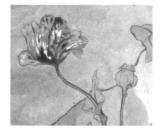

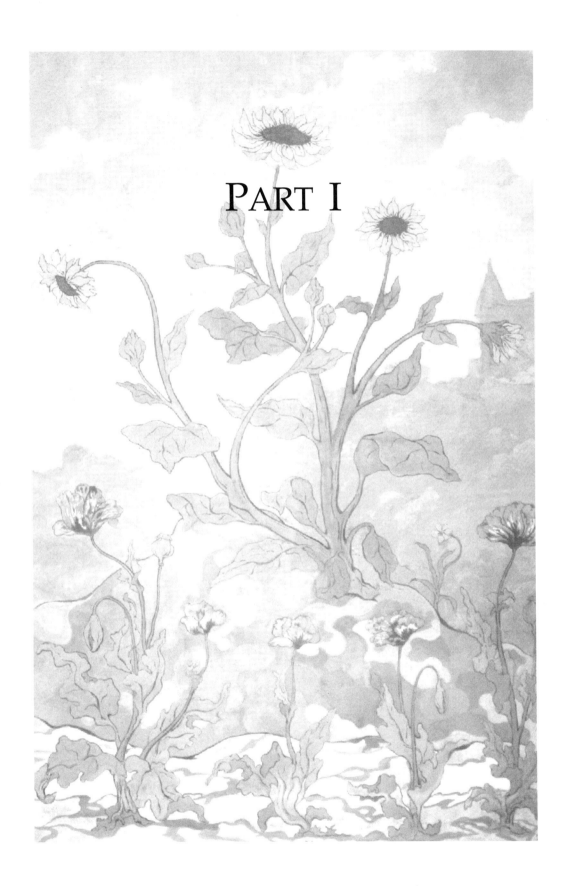

PART I

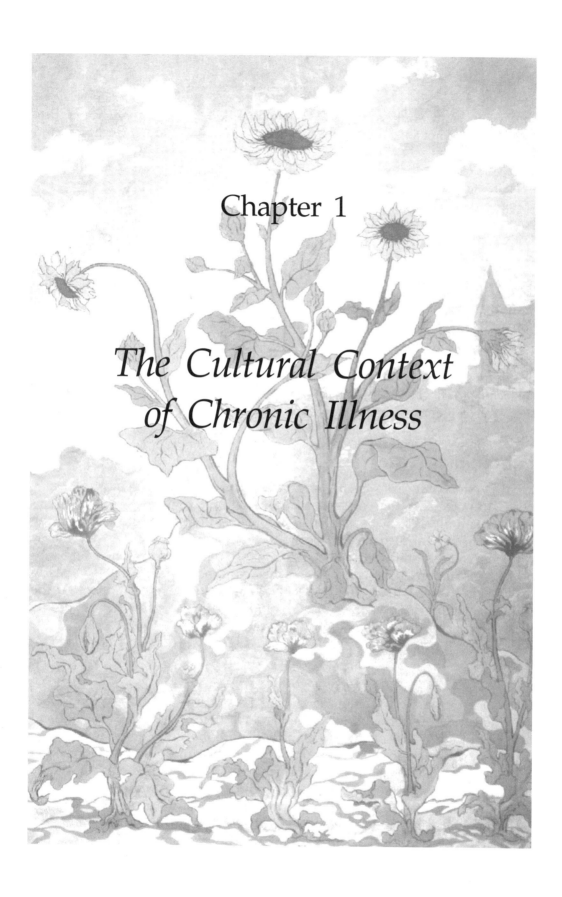

Chapter 1

The Cultural Context
of Chronic Illness

Cultural Context

You don't get sick in a vacuum. You, your family and friends, your co-workers, and your doctors all live in the culture at large. That culture exerts an enormous influence on what everyone thinks about your illness and how they'll treat you. Certain aspects of the general culture will support and help you in your illness. But unfortunately, much of the time the culture is what makes living with your chronic illness difficult. In this chapter I'm going to talk mostly about the negative aspects of the culture but I don't want you to get discouraged. Remember that in part II you are going to learn how to live, work, and interact with people so that you can overcome the problems that the culture so often creates for chronically ill people.

You're probably quite aware of some cultural influences in your life, but like most people, you're probably completely unconscious of many others. Attitudes and influences come to you (and everyone else) from your family, your religion, your ethnic or racial group, your social class, the educational system, the legal system, your workplace, and of course the media. When you're sick, you're most strongly affected by the cultural attitudes of the health-care system. While parts of it can be supportive, you're also constantly subjected to negative influences and effects, even though you may be unaware of them or not realize where they're coming from.

Functions of the Health-Care System

What is the health-care system supposed to do? First and foremost, it's supposed to make sure that you get an up-to-date medical response when you have certain physical or psychological problems. But in American society the health-care system also has an economic function that affects your illness experience very significantly. The system has to pay all its personnel and support its institutions (hospitals, clinics, medical schools, etc.), and it wants to make a profit as well. Finally, the health-care system has an impact on the country's social class system. This, too, can have a major effect on you, particularly if you are poor, female, or a person of color.

Institutions of Care

The most visible parts of the health-care system are the organizations that provide care. You know about hospitals and clinics, with their doctors and nurses. But other, less obvious organizations are those that govern care—the professional associations, government regulatory bodies, the insurance organizations and HMOs, and advocacy groups. In addition, there are all the training and research organizations, including medical schools, universities, government facilities, and for-profit firms working in pharmaceuticals, medical equipment, surgical supplies, etc. And finally, there's probably the most important institution of care of all—your home and family.

Institutional obstacles. You've probably had a few memorable experiences dealing with the physical obstacles that some health-care institutions can present, like when you've tried to park at the hospital or negotiate its bewildering array of corridors. You've probably also run through bureaucratic hassles in which you're asked for guarantees of payment or HMO permission slips while you're desperate to see the doctor or get some lab results. So you know some of the difficulties the health-care system can throw in your way.

Health-care governing bodies. It may not occur to you that the governing bodies of medicine determine whether what's happening to you even qualifies as a disease. They decide if your pain and symptoms are going to be treated as a physical illness, or "just something in your head." In addition, they set the rules for how doctors are supposed to take notes and keep records. If you have a chronic disease you may need to apply for disability, so what your doctor has in his notes and records is vitally important. Governing bodies also determine how doctors are supposed to behave toward you and what they are required to tell you.

Medical schools. The training that doctors and nurses receive makes a big difference in how you experience your illness. Some chronic illnesses are not discussed in medical school, so doctors have to learn about them elsewhere—often from their patients! For the most part, medical students study acute conditions, which have a clear beginning, course, and end or cure. They have little education in the radical differences between how people experience chronic illnesses and how they experience acute illnesses.

Mind-body split. One of the most distorting aspects in medical education is the split between mind and body. This came about approximately 400 years ago, at the birth of modern science. Scientific medicine focused on the physical body because researchers thought it could be measured and quantified objectively. On the other hand, things having to do with the mind depended on subjective, qualitative understanding. The mind was too cloudy and unclear to fit the demands of science. Over time most scientific researchers have recognized that the mind and body are not two separate unrelated systems. The health or illness of an individual inevitably involves a mixture of physical and psychological factors. All the same, scientists, health-care personnel, and the public at large continue to regard clearly physical illnesses with more sympathy. Physical illnesses seem to have external causes and to be more objectively "real." The symptoms of illnesses thought to be psychological seem subjective. People often think that if you have a psychological illness or an illness with a psychological component, you have caused your own disease, demonstrating that you have some sort of character flaw. If your chronic illness is thought to have a psychological cause, then many people (including some doctors) think that you could get better if you wanted to. Some conclude you must therefore be faking, malingering, or simply "bad."

Objective-subjective. Since the scientific revolution, knowledge believed to be objective and technological has come to be valued more than knowledge arrived at subjectively. Certainly objective science has been responsible for enormous advances in the quality of life, but serious realities have been ignored because people denigrate subjectivity and anything assumed to be subjective. Actually, objective thinking is rarely as objective as many scientists claim. The important thing here for anyone with a chronic illness is that most objective, scientific doctors prefer clear physical diseases, with clear external causes, clear courses, and clear outcomes. They may deal poorly with the ambiguities inherent in chronic illnesses.

Research institutions. Most funding that research institutions attract is earmarked to investigate diseases for which they may find cures or for which there is broad social sympathy and media attention. Moreover, because of the social stigma attached to some chronic illnesses and the lack of funds devoted to them, specializing in those diseases isn't very popular. Doctors and researchers are only human, so they usually choose to work in fields that are socially admired and financially rewarding.

Health-insurance companies. The recent changes in medical insurance have brought enormous changes to your experience of health care. You now need to act more like a consumer than a patient when you approach your health-care professionals, and this can be very hard to do when you are scared, confused, and in pain. But you cannot behave as a passive, unquestioning recipient of care anymore. In many cases your health-care provider must now operate as a business person rather than solely as a compassionate health-care professional.

Advocacy groups. Advocacy groups offer you an excellent way to influence and change the health-care system. They not only keep you up to date on the latest advances in your illness, but also lobby legislators to direct funds toward research in your disease and press government regulatory agencies to move important new drugs onto the market.

Your home. Your family and home are often a very mixed environment if you are chronically ill. Every family has developed its own way for thinking about people who are sick, especially if they are members of the family. Your family also has well-established ways for treating family members who are sick. You know these attitudes, even if you and your family never talk about them. Some family ideas about illness come from each family member's individual personality, but most of them come from the family's ethnic, religious, social, educational, and economic background. How chronically ill people are treated in a poor, refugee Cambodian family living in Lawrence, Massachusetts, will be different from how they are treated in a rich Lutheran family in Minneapolis, or a professional black family in San Francisco.

People in the Health-Care System

The health-care system is made up of people as well as organizations. These extend far beyond you, your family, and your doctor. They include nurses and aides, pharmacists and social workers, rehabilitation specialists and psychologists, advocates and standard setters, academics and researchers, members of government agencies and legislators, receptionists and accountants, hospital directors and insurance CEOs. All of these people have an impact on you and, hard as it may be to believe, you have an impact on them. It is also vital to remember that everyone in the health-care system is going to play some other role in the health-care system at another time in their lives. The doctor or the CEO will become a patient, the nurse may become a researcher, and the patient may turn into an advocate who affects the thinking of legislators.

Beliefs, attitudes, norms, and rules in health care. All the people in the health-care system bring their own beliefs and attitudes about health and sickness to the workings of the system. These govern these people's behavior toward the sick, the infirm, and the disabled. Few of these beliefs and attitudes are written down, and sometimes people aren't even aware of what drives their behavior. Some rules and regulations, regarding doctors' behavior for example, are written down, but these are increasingly coming into conflict with others aspects of the changing health-care scene. Some HMOs restrict the time your doctors may spend with you. Contractual relationships between doctors and insurance companies may also limit what your doctors can tell you or how they can treat you.

Invisible attitudes in the health-care system. Invisible attitudes and beliefs within the health-care system concern issues of power and authority, illness etiquette, and care procurement and delivery. It used to be, for example, that doctors had a position of supreme authority. As a patient you were supposed to do what you were told without question. Today your relationship with the doctor is evolving toward more participation on your part, but old attitudes die hard. Some doctors take it as a personal slight and get very annoyed when you ask questions or wish to secure a second opinion.

Invisible attitudes in society at large. People in all parts of society have complicated, conflicting attitudes about illness. These ideas vary enormously depending on each individual's family, religion, ethnic and racial background, economic status, etc. Although American culture offers compassionate ways for reacting to disease and disaster, many people unconsciously or consciously believe that individuals bring illness upon themselves, or that God sends it to them as punishment for bad behavior. This judgmental attitude can make life very difficult if you have a chronic illness. American attitudes toward illness are also affected by old Puritan beliefs that idleness invites the Devil's attention. In the old days, illness or disability could easily seem a sign of the Devil's work. Even the proud notion of the rugged

American individualist who doesn't need help from anyone but who pulls himself up by his own bootstraps can make you seem whiny and feeble in character if you are sick or disabled.

Economic attitudes. Besides regarding illness as a moral issue, some Americans also believe that the sick and disabled put an intolerable strain on the country's economic resources. Although America, the world's leading economic power, offers some of the poorest health-care options of all the industrialized nations, such people believe our country's spending on health care is still excessive. Chronic illnesses never get cured, so money devoted to them particularly angers these critics.

Economic strains of chronic illness. The economic strains of your chronic illness can be particularly cruel in your own family and put enormous stresses on your relationships with family members. This is not a minor concern, but a very important element of living with chronic illness. I will cover this issue thoroughly in part II as I show you how you can handle the issues that come up in each phase of your chronic illness.

Influence of the media. The media play an enormous role in shaping the country's attitudes and opinions. Because of media glamour and power, media pronouncements become powerful myths in the society and are believed implicitly until another story replaces the first. People assume that the media tells the truth. But in fact, television and movies often misrepresent illnesses. They tend to create or expand on generalizations and stereotypes about illness and disability. They draw heavily on current cultural and political trends. What you think is "information" has actually been developed merely to entertain you. The media want to hold your attention so that they can sell you a product, convey a political point of view, or both. How the media represent individuals with breast cancer or chronic fatigue syndrome or Gulf War syndrome shifts with every change in the political and cultural climate.

Positive cultural elements. There are, of course, positive elements in the culture that will support you if you are chronically ill. Many religious institutions have a deep and compassionate commitment to help and care for the sick. Advocacy organizations frequently help organize local support groups and provide information that people can take to their health-care professionals. Community associations, particularly in poor neighborhoods, seek to aid those in need regardless of the reason. And more and more, people who have been hurt or stigmatized by the society for their illness are going public and refusing to be treated that way anymore.

Six Harmful Cultural Factors

There are six cultural factors that dramatically affect the worldview and consequently the behavior of the people in the health-care system. If your health-care professionals do not think about these factors and understand them, then you, your family, and sometimes even the doctors themselves will suffer hurt or trauma.

Intolerance of Suffering

The society we live in can't tolerate suffering. Four hundred years ago when scientists decided that the body and the mind should be separated so that they could pursue measurable, quantitative, objective investigations, they also attempted to separate physical from mental suffering. They thought physical suffering could be relieved as science advanced. But the scientists eventually found that you can't separate physical and mental suffering. Furthermore it's impossible to measure physical suffering objectively. Researchers always had to rely on the reports of the individual who was in pain, and everyone knows that an individual's report is subjective, not scientifically objective. As a practical medical matter, doctors had to deal with these subjective pain reports, but they did not like it and often decided on their own whether the patient's reported pain was physical, and hence legitimate, or mental, and hence suspect.

Characteristics of suffering. Suffering is part of the human condition everywhere. It has certain characteristics:

- It increases in relation to how uncontrollable it is or how uncontrollable you think it will be.

- It increases in relation to how long you think it will last.

- Persistent suffering makes you feel profoundly helpless and hopeless.

- Suffering increases when you're unsure about your future prospects.

- Persistent suffering diminishes your physical, cognitive, and emotional viability, and hence it greatly reduces your sense of self.

- A diminished sense of self causes debilitating grief.

Suffering is perceived as having no value. Most Americans regard suffering as having no positive value whatsoever. It is bad, frightening, and meaningless. If they begin to suffer, they demand immediate, aggressive action to end it. They dislike seeing suffering in others, partly because it makes them unhappy to see others suffer and partly because the suffering of other people reminds them that all life is fragile, and they themselves may suffer in the future.

Suffering causes grief that cannot be expressed. When people are suffering or witnessing the suffering of others, they feel grief and often shame as well. But American society frowns on public expressions of such feelings, especially among men. So sufferers and witnesses alike are forced to push their feelings underground. These suppressed emotions often reemerge in destructive behavior. In other words, you are hurt or traumatized when you're not allowed to express the emotions of grief you feel when you're suffering. Those around you who witness your suffering can also suffer trauma if they can't express their grief.

How health-care professionals protect themselves. Health-care professionals, who have to be around suffering all the time, do exactly what you'd expect to protect themselves. They locate a cause for the suffering as quickly as possible and provide appropriate treatment to end it. If, however, they can't find the cause or if the suffering persists even with treatment, some professionals get frustrated or angry. At this point, rather than admit failure or inadequacy on their part, they may decide that your suffering has a psychological cause, which can imply a character flaw on your part.

Inaccurate reporting. If doctors can't make your suffering go away, they may feel incompetent, and this feeling quickly gets communicated to you. You learn to report only those things that you think the doctor wants to hear. You also figure out that the doctor prefers to hear about physical symptoms. Over time, as you give more and more censored information, the doctor gets a less and less accurate picture of your actual condition.

Iatrogenic trauma. As a consequence of how health-care personnel behave, you may feel worse after going to the doctor. You get confused about what is real. You can't tell if you're sick, well, or just crazy. You don't know whom to trust. You've gone to the doctor for help, for answers, or at least for solace, and you've come away feeling confused, blamed, frightened, and vaguely immoral.

Hiding the truth. At the same time, your family and friends also would rather hear about improvements. They usually think it's not good for you to dwell on negative things. So fearing criticism, rejection, and social abandonment, you learn to censor your experience, skew your medical reporting, and in general misrepresent how you're actually feeling. You begin to pretend to be normal and try to "pass" as healthy. Because this is exhausting, you may decide to avoid intimacy altogether. So you become socially isolated. Marital problems can arise, and you may turn to drugs or alcohol to assuage your pain. You may even contemplate suicide.

Your social contract has been broken. The greatest trauma caused by the culture's intolerance of suffering is the violation of the social contract. You've worked hard to perform as a good partner, parent, worker, and friend. Suddenly you find that something beyond your control has turned you into a second-class citizen who's barely tolerated. Vows that your partner will be loyal "for better or for worse" may become meaningless. The health-care profession, to which you thought you should turn, not only fails to help you, but may even imply that your suffering is your own fault.

Intolerance of Ambiguity

Most people in Western culture are also intolerant of ambiguity. This is an outcome of scientific thinking. People dislike the not-yet-known or the unknowable. They avoid and even fear complexity or chaos. People want issues to be clear and straightforward and solutions to be simple. The primacy of science and technology has contributed to this because science elevates quantitative systems of knowing and simultaneously devalues qualitative and subjective systems of knowing. Anything that isn't observable and measurable is suspect.

Body-mind split. Once again, the body-mind split comes up. Those things related to the physical body are knowable and clear, but anything related to the mind is unknowable, ambiguous, and hence suspect. When health-care professionals can't understand a physical condition, they think by default that it must emerge from the mind. This further contributes to the view that ambiguous situations or problems are somehow dangerous, possibly immoral, and preferably avoided.

Powerlessness. Ambiguity makes you powerless. If you don't know what something is, you can't take action, which makes you feel even more impotent. For some people, diagnosis of even a horrible disease is preferable to an ambiguous condition. Chronic conditions are almost always ambiguous.

Fear of contagion. People are often frightened of the chronically ill simply because their condition is ambiguous. Perhaps you're contagious. This reaction may be an ancient survival instinct, but even when science has clearly identified modes of disease transmission, people still fear contamination. When no one knows where a disease comes from, then perhaps it's easy to catch. If the prognosis of the disease is unclear, who knows what might happen if you got it?

A "just" world. Flooding in to relieve the anxiety caused by ambiguity comes the notion of the "just" world and deserved punishment. People automatically begin to distance themselves from you if you're suffering, especially if the cause is ambiguous. Lots of people have a comforting belief that if they exercise farsighted, protective action, they can avoid personal tragedy. They figure out how they would have avoided your situation, solved it differently, or responded differently. This thinking creates for them a false sense of calm and control over the uncertainty of living. Eventually, it also leads people to blame you for your problems. Perhaps you brought your chronic illness on yourself. Perhaps you're lazy or trying to get out of responsibilities. Perhaps you're being justly punished for something bad you did.

Are you to blame? Like many people suffering a chronic illness, you may come to agree with this notion of guilt. Perhaps you are to blame. Perhaps you deserve what has happened. You feel guilt, depression, and grief, as well as helplessness and confusion. The most serious damage caused the chronically ill by society's intolerance of ambiguity is the open or subtle accusation that the chronically ill are responsible for their condition.

Intolerance of Chronic Illness

Americans are action and achievement oriented. The society prefers acute illnesses because they have a distinct beginning, middle, and end. Even though they disturb personal and organizational output, they are predictable. Chronic illnesses, on the other hand, don't have a distinct beginning, middle, and end, and they're not easily treatable. They run contrary to popular opinion that real medical problems have a single cause and will respond to powerful drugs or quick technological intervention.

People accept only acute conditions. Even when a chronic illness is well understood, it is rarely as well accepted by either health-care professionals or the general public as an acute disease. This is because the nation's whole conception of sickness and health is built on a framework of acute illness. In acute disease, either you are well or you have a specific illness. If you're sick, you either get better on your own, you go to doctors who cure you, or you die. You may get sick again with a different sickness or a different instance of the same disease. But to suffer the ups and downs of a chronic illness tends to try people's patience and understanding.

It is very important to remember that this divided way of thinking about illness as acute or chronic is not a hard fact of science. It is not the same as the distance to the moon or the boiling point of water. It is a social construction—an explanation that the society has made up. Society can change if it wishes.

Drive for cures produces failures. As a consequence of the focus on acute disease, doctors spend their time trying to achieve cures. That is, they try to return you to essentially the same state you were in before the disease. Americans have come to expect cures, especially in the past fifty years with the proliferation of miracle drugs and technological marvels. But if you're chronically ill, you don't get cured. As a result, you and your doctors repeatedly feel like you've both failed. Since everyone—your doctors, family, friends, co-workers—want you to get well, you may try to act as though you've returned to normal. But the strain of acting so counter to reality usually leads to relapse or to social withdrawal.

Absence of chronic treatment methods. There haven't been good treatment methods for the chronically ill in part because doctors have concentrated on acute diseases and because proper treatment seems to involve several different professions. Doctors may not feel professionally responsible for treating what they think of as their patients' mental or social problems, even though these problems are an integral part of chronic illness.

Obsession with illness. If you never get better the way everyone, including yourself, wants you to, you may end up thinking about your illness all the time. Are you a person who has an illness, or is the illness all that you are? No one sees you in any way apart from your illness. Probably the most traumatic effect of society's intolerance of chronic illness is this obsession that patients can have regarding their sickness. It is also an insidious effect, because when you're finally ready to branch out from your preoccupation, everyone you know keeps regarding you solely in terms of your illness.

Current Cultural Perception of Disease

Every illness—TB, atherosclerosis, lupus, or AIDS—is born at a specific time when the culture has certain specific ideas about illness. These ideas are constantly evolving, not simply with regard to particular diseases, but about other kinds of illness as well. Today is not the same health environment as 1950 was. A chronic illness identified tomorrow would appear in a world that has become familiar with AIDS and chronic fatigue syndrome.

Fears of new diseases. When a new illness first appears, most people, even scientists, can be very frightened. They try to avoid anyone who has the disease. As researchers begin to understand the causes and course of an illness, they begin to relax. Although it is serious or even deadly, the disease gradually becomes familiar. People have heard of it, and doctors know how to treat it.

When you contract your illness. At what point in its history you get a disease makes an enormous difference in your experience of it. To contract multiple sclerosis in 1950 was an entirely different experience than getting it today. If you become ill with a disease that has become familiar to the health-care profession and the culture in general, you will tend to be believed as you describe your symptoms and treated with more compassion.

Ill people are outsiders. Regardless of how "acceptable" your disease has become, simply having it marks you as being outside society's primary defining group—the healthy. Indeed, by being different from this basic tribal group, you actually help to define who the healthy are.

Outsiders of any sort, however, tend to arouse suspicion. You may be assigned negative personality characteristics, especially when you're talking with health professionals or claims managers. They may suspect you of malingering, of not wanting to pull your own weight. They may presume you are mentally ill because you can't meet the demands of ordinary life. Or they may simply judge you to be a bad person who's trying to manipulate the health-care system for some inappropriate end.

Not surprisingly, such attitudes can make you feel socially awkward. You may feel ashamed, and your self-esteem can plummet as a result. If you're like most chronically ill individuals, you may feel truly different from everyone else for the first time in your life. Maybe you really are the damaged goods, the outcast, that society says you are.

Illness Enculturation Process

Once health-care professionals have identified a new disease, they assess it, research it, and learn how to treat it. As they become familiar with the illness, the society at large simultaneously begins to learn about it and evaluate it. Eventually the disease and society's assessment of it becomes a part of everyday social reality. This process is the disease enculturation process.

Social evaluations of illnesses. At the start, just about everyone fears a new disease and avoids anyone afflicted with it, as happened with AIDS. As they are enculturated, however, most diseases become acceptable. Forty years ago, people believed you could "catch" cancer, and cancer victims were shunned. Today most cancer victims are regarded with sympathy. But schizophrenia is still considered an unacceptable, morally tainted illness. Some chronic illnesses like lupus or multiple sclerosis are well along in the enculturation process, so they are reasonably acceptable to society. Others, like fibromyalgia or Gulf War syndrome, are still regarded with deep suspicion by many people, including health-care professionals.

Absence of language or models. At the beginning of an illness, no one—neither doctors nor patients—has the language to describe accurately what is happening. There are not even adequate metaphors. The language for saying what's wrong in any disease is very conventional and develops over time. At the beginning of an illness, doctors also have no models for assessing the symptoms, let alone treating the illness. Usually they try to treat a new illness in the way that they would treat something similar that they're familiar with. But with chronic conditions, such treatments, which are almost always based on acute illness models, are frequently unsatisfactory.

Not pure science. Determining the authenticity of a new illness, which is part of the enculturation process, is never a matter of "pure" science. Political and economic issues always cloud the investigation. Research funds or social support may be denied, and in addition, subtle negative attitudes from the culture at large may affect anyone, even scientific researchers.

During the enculturation period, the media may say whatever they like about the new condition. They can make any judgments they want about people who say they are sick with the illness. Given the predispositions of the culture, the media usually reacts with disbelief that the condition is an actual physical illness. They tend to ridicule the condition and condemn people who claim to be suffering from it. If you're suffering with this condition, you're obviously going to be hurt by these misrepresentations.

Impact on patients. How safe you feel and how much trust you place in the community is going to depend a lot on when in the illness enculturation process you are diagnosed. If your disease is in its infancy, you will suffer greater powerlessness and more trauma than if you are diagnosed later in the process. With an enculturated disease, you and your family have language to use with doctors and others. Moreover, people will have some awareness of and perhaps even sympathy for your problem.

Influence of the Media

Public judgments. The media function as a forum for public opinion and judgment in addition to conveying information. They popularize professional medical findings, but often present the material without conveying any indication of how tentative and liable to revision some findings are. Because the media want drama or entertainment that will sell goods, they are not above manipulating information to the greatest dramatic effect. The media also exert an enormous influence by creating and reinforcing social stereotypes and cultural prejudices. They publicly determine the worth of different roles in society, and they organize public ridicule or support.

Invasion of privacy. You or your family may easily find your illness appearing as a headline horror story in a supermarket tabloid. Or a TV movie-of-the-week may present a drama that purports to detail exactly what you've experienced. Or a celebrity may be diagnosed with your illness, thereupon setting off a frenzy of stories about your condition. Even if the media treat your condition with sympathy, your privacy is invaded. Suddenly all your friends and co-workers have access to intimate details of your illness, which you may not really want to share with them. You may not have even experienced aspects of the disease that are dramatized, but people will be convinced that you must have. Moreover, the sympathy demonstrated in one media story can quickly turn to ridicule, scorn, or anger in another. Such public judgment of your condition and your character may make you withdraw even further from friends and acquaintances. Even if you have had strong social connections prior to your illness, after you get sick these connections almost always erode.

Moving Out of the Negative Context

In this chapter we've looked at the cultural content of chronic illness, particularly in the health-care system. We've examined the institutions of care and the people in the health-care system. We've looked at factors, particularly ideas and attitudes, that affect how the health-care system operates. Sometimes these attitudes are conscious, but often they're not. We then noted six cultural factors that almost always have harmful effects on those with chronic illnesses. These include societal intolerance of suffering and of ambiguity and intolerance of chronic as opposed to acute illness. We called attention to the current cultural perception of disease in general, to the illness enculturation process, and to the enormous influence of the media. It can seem like a very discouraging prospect.

But you can move out of this negative world. In the next chapter, I'll give you a general overview of the four-phase model, and then I'll tell you the story of Betty, an individual with MS. Her physical, psychological, and social experiences as she goes through the phase process will show you how she learns to achieve a full, manageable, meaningful life, even with her illness.

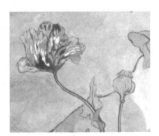

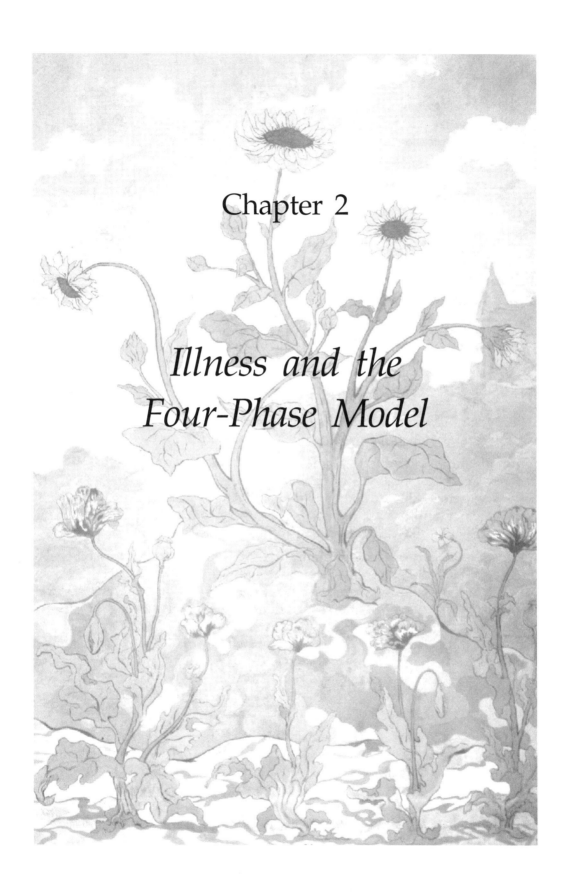

Chapter 2

*Illness and the
Four-Phase Model*

Phase Model Helps in Any Chronic Illness

No matter what particular illness you have, you can improve the quality of your life if you learn about the phases that people with chronic illness experience. You may have an illness like diabetes, rheumatoid arthritis, multiple sclerosis, lupus, chronic fatigue syndrome, and so on. Most of the medical profession regard these illnesses as chronic physiological illnesses. Or you may have a disease like HIV/AIDS, cancer, or have had a stroke. These diseases have responded to treatment so well that people now experience them as chronic rather than acute diseases. Or you may suffer from conditions such as addiction, alcoholism, post-traumatic stress syndrome, or situations involving intractable pain. These conditions also respond well to phase-model assessment and treatment. The reason is because all these conditions have important factors in common. Using the phase model will help you understand what is happening to you over time as you live with your illness. It will also help you make meaningful improvements in your treatment and your life situation.

Embedded Systems

When you're sick, your illness is not something isolated and separate. It's part of several embedded systems.

Body-mind integrated system. I believe that all illnesses have physical and psychological components. In chronic illness especially, it is absolutely necessary to treat both the body and the mind simultaneously. The two always work together, and to treat only one will never produce long-lasting, beneficial results. You, like all individuals, are a combined mind-body system.

Patient as part of family, community, workplace systems. I also believe that no one is simply an individual mind-body system, but that you are also part of a family. Your family may or may not be your biological relatives and your relatives by marriage. It also includes anyone whom you regard as your "family." These may be friends, neighbors, members of your church, or anyone who is important to you the way that people traditionally think family members are. You are also part of a community (or many communities), and you may be part of a workplace, too. Any illness you have, especially a chronic illness, is going to affect how you live in all these worlds, and it is also going to affect the worlds themselves.

Clinician as part of a patient-family system. Your doctor or clinician also becomes part of the many systems you live in. Your doctor will affect you and all those around you, and you and your family will also affect your doctor. All the systems that you live in can reduce, magnify, or sometimes even create symptoms in you and in those around you. Because of this, you need to have assessment and treatment of your illness that takes all these systems into consideration.

False Oppositions

Body-mind. I've already mentioned how the distinction made between mind and body creates a false opposition. What happens in your body affects your mind and emotions. Your mind and emotions affect what happens in your body. It is very hard to figure out whether the mind and emotions started something or the body did, and which came first has very little bearing on how you need to treat a condition once it has begun. You need to treat both mind and body.

Objective-subjective. The division between mind and body helped to foster the notion that there was a sharp distinction between objective, rational, materialist thinking and subjective, intuitive perception. Because scientists were thought to engage in objective thinking that produced all sorts of useful knowledge, the society came to place the highest value on it. Subjective understanding was considered less valuable. Actually, so-called objective thinking is filled with subjective attitudes, and many aspects of living in the world cannot be investigated with the tools of objective rationalism.

Professional-personal. Another fallout from the development of science, especially in medicine, was how society came to regard doctors. When they were doing their job, doctors were meant to behave as purely objective professionals, even though they were subjective individuals in their private lives. To this day many doctors are trained to hold their personal selves apart when practicing medicine. If patients or the conditions patients suffer arouse feelings in doctors, the doctors are said to be experiencing "countertransference." They are strongly encouraged to overcome such feelings. Not surprisingly, if your doctors are successful in quashing their feelings, they may appear to you as cold, distant, impersonal, and unfeeling. In the hands of such professionals, you may well think that you aren't getting the kind of "care" that you want. In the Phase Model, health-care professionals learn to use their personal feelings and perceptions to improve their treatment of you and strengthen their relationship with you.

Clinician-patient. Another false opposition that has grown up is the one that says doctors are different from patients. Unfortunately, many of us, including doctors, have come to believe this. Because doctors appear to hold the power of life and death, it is easy to suppose that they are really a different sort of creature than you are. Obviously they're trained in information that you don't know, but they're not intrinsically different from you. They are human beings. They are subject to all the same joys and problems that you are. If you come to think doctors have supreme powers, you'll be very disappointed if they don't cure you. And doctors who think they are godlike tend to become very disappointed in the patients they cannot cure. Rather than admit inability, they may decide that it is the patient who is making a cure impossible.

Illness as unusual vs. illness as normal life. In America, most people think that being sick or having an illness is unusual. They think that the normal state of affairs is to be healthy. Of course, everyone would rather be healthy than sick. But illness is a regular part of normal life, just as death is, and refusing to acknowledge that fact will not make illness go away. As more and more people come to have some kind of chronic illness—and the American Medical Association says that now almost half of the population have a chronic illness—it's going to be harder to ignore just how normal illness is. Perhaps this will eventually lead to beneficial changes in social attitudes.

Static vs. dynamic disabilities. The society has come to have entirely new attitudes toward people with disabilities, but it still lacks awareness that many illnesses are disabling. It also lacks knowledge that disabilities can change and that a disability may not be obviously visible. Most people tend to think of disability in terms of someone with a *static* condition, sitting in a wheelchair. But if you have a chronic illness, your disabilities can get worse or better in a cyclical, *dynamic*, way. In addition, many of your disabilities may not be visually obvious at all. You may look well, but be suffering from such debilitating exhaustion that you cannot walk unaided.

Acute vs. chronic illness. Modern Western medicine has, throughout its history, focused on *acute* diseases, which hopefully have a single clear cause, a specific onset, identifiable symptoms, usually a single treatment, and ultimately a cure. People didn't used to think very much about *chronic* illnesses because most people didn't live long enough for them to be commonplace. Now that Americans are living longer, more and more people are coming to suffer from chronic illnesses. Some are even acute diseases that have responded so well to treatment that people who would have died in the past now live for long periods of time with the illness. Many chronic diseases are not like acute diseases. They do not have single, clear causes, specific onsets, or linear courses. You have remission of symptoms and then relapses. Your condition is constantly changing over time, and symptoms that bother you enormously may not be present on the specific day when you actually have a doctor's appointment. These illnesses are often diagnosed when you accumulate a certain number of specific symptoms. But doctors have to rely on your reporting of these symptoms, so it may be easy for them to assume that your mind is creating your problem or some of the symptoms. Chronic illnesses can rarely be treated completely by drugs or physical therapy. Either may work for a time to help specific symptoms, but then the illness may manifest itself in other symptoms for which there are no drugs. Moreover, as your symptoms change, you often need not continue with treatments prescribed for you earlier.

Economics and chronicity. So treatment of your chronic illness is constantly shifting, and successful treatment depends on your having a strong, trusting relationship with your health-care professional. But nowadays the economics of medicine works against this. The health organizations that most doctors work for limit the time they can spend with you and so they may not get the full, shifting picture of your condition. You may also find that your insurance will not permit you to see all the specialists who may be pertinent to your illness.

Traumatization of the Chronically Ill

Work ethic. The culture is built around an idealized work ethic in which healthy, productive people are considered socially useful and valuable, while people who are very young, very old, differently abled, or infirm may be loved and indulged but are not seen as contributing to the good of society. Since people with chronic illness are often unable to work at their former pace, and since they often have few outward signs of illness, they are often perceived as trying to escape from doing their fair share. It's important to remember that as a member of the culture, you very likely think this way, too. You may not care for yourself the way you could because you aren't contributing to society the way you believe that you should.

Traumas of the chronically ill. Quite apart from your painful symptoms, you and those around you can get hurt by your chronic illness. Whether you suffer any of these hurts and how much you suffer depends in part on the severity of your illness. These hurts or traumas occur in a number of different ways.

- **Illness onset.** The realization that something is very wrong with you can deeply hurt you in and of itself.

- **Family response.** Your family may not be able to adjust to the changes your chronic illness brings to your life, and their reactions can hurt you.

- **Society's response.** Your friends, your co-workers, and the society at large can hurt you because they are afraid of your disease, misunderstand it, or feel awkward around the changed you. In some cases you may suffer from bias fostered by the media and lose your job or housing opportunities, your financial credit, your friendships, even your spouse.

- **Unrelated traumas.** You may have had serious traumas before becoming sick or have other unrelated traumas which occur while you are sick, such as a death in the family or experience of a natural disaster, a car accident, military service in a war zone, etc. These traumas will have an additional impact on your chronic illness.

- **Clinically caused traumas.** Iatrogenic traumas are hurts which the health-care profession cause you. When you are disbelieved by a doctor or treated as though your chronic illness is simply a psychological problem, you can suffer a clinically caused trauma.

- **Vicarious trauma.** Those who live, love, and work with you can also be traumatized because of your illness. They suffer from all of the traumas listed above. Doctors and other health-care professionals can also suffer vicarious traumas in relation to your illness, especially within the profession. Doctors who treat patients or diseases that the society doesn't value may suffer both professionally and financially.

Integration Assumption

Unlike the traditional medical approach, the four-phase model does not assume that you will eventually be cured. Instead it seeks to integrate your illness into a different but meaningful life. If you do not achieve illness integration, the chances are that you will suffer repeated failures at each relapse and change in your illness. The four-phase model pursues specific treatments to eliminate or reduce your disease symptoms, but unlike the traditional medical approach, it also uses palliation as an *active* treatment option. *Palliation* is the reduction of suffering. Often health-care workers believe they are providing palliation when they reduce physical symptoms. But true palliation actually includes the relief of suffering in the psychological and social aspects of the patient's life as well as in the physical aspects. In the four-phase model, palliation includes interventions to improve your psychological and social well-being, and when possible to improve the situation for those around you. The phase model also encourages you, your family, and your health-care provider to work together. Medical specialists in this model don't treat from outside but become part of a holistic system. They become co-conspirators, if you will, with you and your family.

The Four Phases

I have used the term "phase" rather than "stage" because stages imply a progression that only goes forward. The phase model recognizes that you are liable to be thrown back into earlier phases when new and unforeseen crises occur in your life. You may also experience aspects of two different phases at the same time. If, however, you work through the phases once, you have the skills and the knowledge to take you through the processing sequence more quickly so that you arrive more speedily at integration of the new experience. It's also important to remember that you experience each phase in three different areas. Changes occur in your *physical* life, in your *psychological* life, and in your *social and work* life. As you read this book, you will see what happens specifically in each phase in each area and what you can do to help yourself.

Phase One: Crisis

Phase one is characterized by crisis and chaos. In this phase you move from the actual onset of your illness to an emergency stage that usually forces you to seek some sort of relief. Most people desperately seek a medical diagnosis and treatment of the problem. But others may look for spiritual help. Still others may simply try to ease the pain they feel by alcohol or drugs.

Your task—and that of your family and doctor—during phase one is to deal with the immediate hurts or traumas of your new illness.

Phase Two: Stabilization

In phase two, you have reached a plateau of symptoms, and because they stay more or less the same, they become familiar. You begin to think that maybe you're getting a little better. You still continue to experience a lot of chaos, however. You usually keep trying to behave as you did before you got sick, and this attempt frequently leads to relapses. These are very upsetting and feel like personal failures. But because a certain amount of the time you feel like you can manage, you keep trying to find a way to return to your old life. The task of phase two is to begin to stabilize and restructure your life patterns and perceptions.

Phase Three: Resolution

Phase three may bring a plateau of symptoms or you may have relapses. But at this point you've learned how your illness behaves and how the world responds to it. You've also finally learned that you can't be the person that you used to be before you got ill. This can be a devastating perception, one that can makes you experience a "dark night of the soul." Your task during phase three is to develop a new, authentic self and to begin to locate a personally meaningful philosophy to live by.

Phase Four: Integration

In phase four, you may experience a plateau of symptoms or periodic relapses, but you're now able to integrate parts of your old self from before the illness with the person you are now. Your task in phase four is to continue to find ways to express your new "personal best," to reintegrate or form new supportive networks of family and friends, to find appropriate employment if you are able to work, or other vocations or activities, and to locate your illness experience within a larger philosophical or spiritual framework. In the most total integration, you arrive at a new, whole, complete life, of which illness is only one part, even if it is an important part.

Betty's Story: a Case History

One of the best ways to get an overall picture of the four-phase model is to examine one person's experience. Betty's story shows you how one person feels in each phase, what she does, how others around her behave, and what her health-care professionals do. Betty is not a real person, but her experiences are a composite of real experiences.

Before starting, however, I want to mention something that has probably already occurred to you. Illness comes to people who are growing and changing just as everyone does during their lifetimes. Young children become adolescents, people seek out partners and some have children, adults seek employment or careers and then change positions or careers, adults care for elderly family members and prepare for their own retirement. Crises that are part and parcel of life's developmental processes may occur at the very same time that your illness occurs, making it hard to tell sometimes what is related to the illness and what is related to, say, the death of a parent. Betty's illness occurred when she was a young married, working woman with two school-aged children.

In addition, you, Betty, and everyone else has a basic physical and mental constitution. Some perfectly healthy people are basically energetic and need little sleep, while others who are just as healthy tire more easily and require lots of rest. Some healthy people are very relaxed and assured emotionally, and they do not get upset easily. Others, who are equally healthy, are nervous, prone to emotional outbursts, and easily distressed. When considering how you or anyone else responds to the experience of chronic illness, you need to think about your basic physical and emotional constitution. You need to consider what you were usually like, both physically and emotionally, before you got sick. Betty had a pretty average physical constitution, neither wildly energetic nor easily tired. Emotionally she was quite hardy, with strong reserves of patience.

Here is Betty's story.

Betty's Phase One

Betty's a married woman in her late thirties. She has two children; Lisa, aged 13, and Michael, aged 11. Betty's husband, Bob, is a computer hardware troubleshooter. He often has to work out of town for one or two weeks at a time. Betty works part-time at a bank in the suburb where the family lives.

Physical aspect. Over the past several weeks, Betty's been increasingly distracted by a number of physical symptoms that are beginning to frighten her because they interfere with her life and her work. She's always tired—in fact, she's exhausted most of the time. But what seems very strange to her is that she sometimes has trouble walking. Her vision also seems blurry. Betty's never had more than the occasional cold, so she rarely goes to the doctor. But she thinks her tiredness is probably not very different from what a lot of her friends feel. They're all working, and many are also mothers. So she just keeps trying to carry on with her regular activities, snatching whatever moments she can to nap or at least rest.

Betty's just entering phase one. She's in a *coping* stage. Even though she doesn't feel well much of the time, she's generally able to push her symptoms out of her consciousness and to continue her regular activities. Many people with chronic conditions are able to cope for a long period of time.

Eventually, however, Betty's condition gets so bad that she can't ignore it, and she enters the *onset* stage. For many chronic patients a particular incident like a flu virus or a car accident triggers onset, but Betty simply feels worse and worse and is able to do less and less. When she realizes one day that she can't walk up a full flight of stairs, she goes to see the doctor.

Her doctor listens to Betty describe her symptoms and gives her a quick physical. They talk a bit about her situation at work and at home. The doctor tells Betty that she has nothing physically wrong with her. What with her job and family life, it sounds as though stress may be causing her difficulties. He also thinks that she is mildly depressed, but not enough to require medication. The doctor recommends that Betty relax, try to get enough sleep, cut back at work, and perhaps join an exercise class to help relieve her stress. Chronically ill individuals, especially women, are often told that they are actually suffering from depression.

Betty wants to follow the doctor's suggestions, but she doesn't dare cut back on work because the family needs her income. And she can't see how to fit an exercise class into her already tight schedule. Her symptoms get worse. She now has trouble driving, and sometimes can barely figure out how to get home. Even her co-workers are beginning to notice her difficulty walking, and she's extremely fatigued all the time. Betty's now entering the *acute emergency* stage. This stage can last for days, weeks, or months for many chronic illness patients, depending on the severity of the illness and the quality of their personal and health-care support.

Betty goes back to the doctor, who now orders a complete physical. For months she's examined and tested. But it's a full year before she gets a tentative diagnosis of multiple sclerosis. Even now, the doctors aren't really sure it's MS. Not all doctors agree on the factors determining MS, and some of Betty's tests are ambiguous. Nevertheless, having a diagnosis, even a tentative one, makes an enormous difference to Betty. She finally has a way to understand and describe her experiences to herself and others.

Psychological aspect. During Betty's long coping and onset stage, when she doesn't know what's going on, she denies to herself and others that anything is wrong. This denial is, after all, one way to cope. Denial comes into play even more strongly after her doctor tells her that she's mildly depressed and suffering from the stress of a modern woman's life.

Like all people, while Betty was growing up she created two selves, a private one and a public one. Like everyone, Betty reveals her private self only to the people she's most intimate with and whom she trusts completely. As Betty's physical condition continues to deteriorate, however, she finds that she can't always control her private emotions and they break through inappropriately in public. One day at a staff meeting, Betty suddenly bursts into tears, embarrassing herself, her superior, and her co-workers. Betty's never been the sort of person who cries in public. She is greatly ashamed of herself and begins to wonder what could possibly be wrong with her. During phase one, many chronically ill individuals begin to experience shame and self-hatred for their loss of psychological self-control.

Betty's shame and self-hatred occur at the same time that she's feeling increased fear and despair. Maybe she's really dying or losing her mind. She knows she feels terrible physically and is getting worse, but maybe something's also wrong with her mind. It's important to remember that at this point no one's labeled Betty's situation yet. No one knows what's going on. At this point, most chronically ill individuals receive conflicting advice and assessments from their family, friends, and medical contacts. The people in Betty's life who know that something is wrong attempt to find explanations for her condition and suggest how she can improve her situation. Her family and friends base their suggestions on personal experiences or information they've gotten from a variety of sources, including other people and stories in the media. These are often unreliable and they often contradict each other. Betty's health-care professionals are trying to arrive at a thoughtful diagnosis of her condition, but they've reached only the most preliminary conclusions, which may make their treatments ineffective.

Betty feels increasingly isolated because she's afraid of what's happening and of what other people will think of her. She's particularly afraid to talk to the one person who used to be closest to her, Bob. Betty and Bob have already been having some marital difficulties. They've fought over money and the amount of time Bob spends away from home. Betty feels that Bob gets out of his fair share of home and child care duties. She can't quit her job to stay home full-time because they need her salary. And anyway, she likes her job, which she does very well. She's gotten a lot of praise at work, and she and Bob both think that she may get a promotion. The new position would bring in more money, but Betty will have to work full-time.

Because of her pain, her fears, her lack of useful information about her condition, and her growing isolation, Betty begins to suffer mood swings. Half the time she's in tears and the other half she's furious. At first Bob tried to be sympathetic, but now he's getting annoyed. The children act scared of her and disappear whenever possible. Even Betty's co-workers find her snappish and distracted, where she used to be pleasant and cooperative.

Social and work aspects. Many of Betty's psychological reactions result directly from what's happening in her social and work life. During the coping and onset stages, Betty's family, friends, and co-workers respond in various ways to what they see of her experiences. While she's in denial about anything being wrong, they notice only that she's tired a lot of the time and perhaps missing work. For a while they are sympathetic. She's a hard worker, and the women at least know how hard it is to juggle a job, home, and children. As Betty accomplishes less and misses more work, however, even her female co-workers become critical. They have difficult lives, too, but they come to work and they accomplish their assigned tasks.

Betty's children think that she acts strange. She doesn't behave like the mother they're used to. Bob finds her unpredictable and emotionally extreme. He's used to hearing Betty say she's tired, but when she complains about blurred vision and trouble with walking, Bob gets genuinely worried and wants her to go to the doctor. The doctor's diagnosis of stress seems reasonable to Bob. He makes an effort to help more by staying in town or taking only short jobs away from home. But that can't go on forever, and Betty doesn't seem to change. He thinks she could do a lot more if she tried, but she seems just to complain or sleep.

During the acute emergency stage, while Betty's being examined and tested extensively, Bob sometimes wonders whether anything is actually wrong with her. Maybe it's all in her head. Some of her co-workers feel that way, too. Maybe Betty is having a kind of nervous breakdown. Actually Betty feels that way sometimes, too.

Finally, Betty gets her diagnosis, however tentative, of MS. Although this gives her the relief of a name and an explanation, she now finds that the illness has put her squarely on the forefront of a cultural debate. What is chronic illness? Are the people who say they are suffering from chronic illness actually sick with genuine disease, deserving of help and sympathy, or are just they faking, either consciously or unconsciously, and trying to get out of their responsibilities? Some of Betty's friends and co-workers, even some of the health-care personnel she sees, regard her negatively. For the first time in her life, she begins to experience social rejection. She quickly becomes very cautious about expressing her fears or revealing her pain because she doesn't want people to back away from her. She tends to tell people, even her doctor, only what she thinks they want to hear. Not only is she afraid of other people now, but her physical condition itself interferes with her reaching out socially. Increasingly, she is isolated as a sufferer within her disease.

Unfortunately, Betty's home life was stressed prior to the onset of her illness. And her illness has made the situation worse. At work, Betty's immediate supervisor is very sympathetic, because the supervisor's sister has a chronic illness called fibromyalgia. The supervisor has a good grasp of Betty's problems and wants to help. However, upper levels of management think that Betty should probably be replaced. On the medical front, Betty's primary physician has become very involved with her case and would like to spend more time on it, but the HMO for which he works permits only fifteen minutes per patient visit. The doctor can't spend the time he would like talking with Betty. He has to focus on testing her physical symptoms, the only ones the HMO regards as "real," and will pay for. The doctor can't explore in depth how Betty's feeling or how she's coping with the whole illness experience.

During phase one, the sick individual is hurt or traumatized by the physical, psychological, and social impact of the chronic illness. But in addition, the individual's family, friends, co-workers, and caregivers can experience shock, disbelief, sometimes revulsion, and then alterations in their life or work patterns when the individual's illness enters the acute emergency stage. As a result, these others can be vicariously traumatized. This usually causes them to queue up along a continuum that extends from support for the individual to suspicion that the individual is malingering. Because some of the responses are very negative, or even stigmatizing, they can cause secondary traumatization in the chronically ill individual.

Betty's Phase Two

During phase two, Betty attempts to create order out of chaos. Her physical symptoms stabilize. They don't disappear, but she reaches a plateau of sorts. She begins to recognize a pattern to her physical condition, and because of this she can orient herself. She knows that if she climbs a set of stairs in the morning, she will not be able to do it later in the day. If she drives for more than ten or fifteen minutes, she will become fatigued and then confused about how to get where she is going. Although life is very difficult, Betty has identified a set of parameters around which she can function. Her health-care professionals discuss a few of these parameters with her, but for the most part Betty discovers them on her own. To some extent, her newfound knowledge also orients the people around her.

Physical aspects. During phase two, Betty suffers two physical relapses, during which her symptoms suddenly become more severe. For one episode her doctor puts her on steroids. Both times she eventually returns to a plateau of stabilized symptoms that she can negotiate.

Psychological aspects. Unlike many people with chronic illness, Betty has gotten a diagnosis. At first this gives her an enormous sense of relief. Finally she has an explanation for why she has difficulty walking, why her vision has deteriorated, why she becomes so fatigued and confused, and why she has such extreme mood swings. She has been freed from some of the ambiguity, uncertainty, and chaos of her situation. Her uncertainties also lessen as she begins to recognize her own symptom pattern. Diagnosis also gives her a way to learn about her condition so that she can exert a bit of control over her life again. She reads everything she can about MS and seeks out other people with MS so that she can discuss her situation in a supportive setting.

But Betty quickly learns that the diagnosis does not explain how her illness started or what is going to happen in the future, so ambiguity returns. No one seems to know what to do to cure her. No one can make her symptoms stop, and no one seems willing or able to tell her how she can live her life under these new conditions.

Betty has already accumulated some experiences of disbelief, rejection, stigmatization, and even iatrogenic traumatization, so she's become very cautious. She's learned to censor what she says and to whom. Betty engages in "passing" for well.

Like most people in this country, Betty grew up believing that if she worked very hard and told the truth, everything would come out all right in her life. But here she is, working extremely hard to get better, telling the truth when she talks to family members, friends, and clinicians, and yet a lot of the time she finds a significant number of people don't understand in the slightest. In fact, she sometimes gets blamed for her condition.

To avoid this secondary wounding, Betty has the fairly healthy reaction of withdrawing from those social contacts. In their place, she tries to locate people like herself, people with MS or advocating for those with MS. They will not hurt her, and they will understand her situation. Betty continues to read up on her condition and seeks other sources of emotional support to make up for the losses she has suffered.

Because her medical outcome is uncertain and Betty still believes that a cure must be a possibility, she suspects that her health-care professionals aren't up to dealing with her problem. She collects the names of other doctors and goes through a period of "doctor-hopping," hoping to find better treatment and a cure. This behavior upsets her primary care physician, who finds this behavior unhelpful.

In fact, Betty's searching shows that she has enough ego strength, now that her symptoms have plateaued, to feel she can assert some control over her life. She's repairing some of the extensive ego loss that occurred during phase one. Her behavior is part of a natural seeking process that occurs in phase two. It's really an expression of hope.

Because Betty finds little guidance and meets with confusing responses and occasionally even outright hostility as she tries a number of doctors, she tries alternative treatment. A practitioner of shiatsu massage listens to her with enormous empathetic patience. Betty's cousin urges her to try acupuncture. A co-worker swears that a complicated vitamin and supplement regime returned her bedridden niece to full functioning and could do the same for Betty.

Physically, Betty doesn't know what she can and can't do. She looks like she's returned to "normal," a false appearance that Betty helps to create by her "passing" behavior. So she's being encouraged, even urged, by her family, friends, and employer to return to her former roles and schedules. But Betty can't do this without serious problems. She has trouble getting up in the morning. Her husband has to make the children's school lunches. She can no longer be on committees at work, since she can hardly keep up with her regular obligations. She feels like a small child just beginning to learn how to get about in the world around her. Nothing about her body or emotions or mind acts the way it used to, and yet she keeps trying to behave as though she were the person she used to be. Despite her efforts, Betty fails daily at what she attempts. As a result she feels guilty and ashamed every day. As time goes on, she feels more and more worthless.

Social and work aspects. Betty has growing conflicts with her family, friends, and some care providers as they lose patience with her failure to "get back to normal." Although she has a diagnosis, the treatment she receives does not produce rapid improvement. During her first relapse, when she had significant difficulty walking, Betty's doctor put her on a course of prednisone. She improved, but she still has periodic difficulties. The persistence of her symptoms frustrates everyone. Bob finally tells her that she's not the person he married and this isn't the life he signed up for. She's got to change or their marriage is over. Betty can tell that her co-workers are annoyed and believe that she could function a lot better if she just pulled herself together and put her mind on the job. Betty knows that some people think she isn't trying hard enough. To make matters worse, a close friend with deep religious convictions has urged Betty to pray, saying that if Betty has a sincere desire to get better and asks for God's help, God will cure her. Betty doesn't share her friend's convictions, but deep inside she fears that maybe she's sick because she somehow offended God.

As Betty goes through cycles of physical relapse and remission, all the people in her life experience them as well. They become as exhausted by the process as Betty does. They are traumatized, just as she is. Bob has lost the wife he married and the life he had. Their son, Michael, has always liked school and done well, but now his grades begin to suffer. Lisa behaves badly at home and has taken up with a rough crowd at school. Betty wonders if these behaviors are just a part of adolescence, or if Lisa and Michael are reacting to her health problems and her squabbles with Bob over money, the division of labor at home, and her condition?

Betty's family isn't mean-spirited. They're sad and scared to see this person who is very important to them suffer pain, confusion, and unhappiness. Outside the house they suffer a kind of guilt by association. Lisa's friends sometimes treat her as though she's as weird as her mother. Lisa once saw one of them imitate for the others the way her mother sometimes walks. Bob's boss is clearly concerned whether Bob will be able to fulfill his job obligations, given the demands of Betty's illness. Some people wonder if what she has is really MS and if it's catching. Just for safety's sake, some tend to keep their distance.

Because people in phase two so often try and fail to return to "normal," it's not unusual for either the chronically ill or those around them to turn to alcohol or drugs. People in the sick person's social network may avoid or sometimes even abuse the chronically ill individual. Any of these factors or even a totally new factor can produce a new crisis in the chronically ill person, which sends them right back to phase one. In Betty's life, Bob's mother dies and the entire family has to deal with that trauma. Later, Betty has a high fever during a bout with flu, which triggers her second severe relapse.

Without informed guidance, many chronically ill people get caught in a repeating loop of phase one and phase two. Each new crisis produces new wounding and secondary wounding. With luck, following each crisis the sick person manages to arrive at a plateau of manageable symptoms. But the next crisis can send the whole system into chaos again. Some people, particularly those on the margins of society with almost no sources of support, never escape phase one. They are buffeted from crisis to crisis, some relieved only by alcohol and drugs. These individuals often lose everything they have had—their jobs, their families, their homes—and some become homeless street people simply because they are sick and have not received the care and help they need.

Betty's not in that position. She has some warm and loyal friends. Her supervisor persuades the bank management to let Betty take a position with fewer hours. And a new nurse practitioner in Betty's doctor's office becomes involved in helping Betty manage her MS. She builds a team to work on Betty's problem. While the nurse practitioner monitors Betty's physical protocols, she refers Betty to a social worker who can help Betty deal with issues relating to her work, her family, and her friends.

Phase Three

In phase three, Betty enjoys long periods of stabilized symptoms, sometimes even improvement, but she still has relapses. Most of these are simply in the nature of her illness. As Betty comes to understand that her condition is chronic and perpetually ambiguous, she lets go of her search for a cure. Instead, she tries to build a new life that makes room for her illness.

Physical aspects. Twice in phase two, Betty suffered severe relapses that came about in part because she repeatedly tried to do all the things she could before she got sick. During that time she wanted to be her former self, and everyone around her wanted her to be that person, too. But repeated relapses taught Betty that she cannot sustain the roles that she had always thought she would fulfill as spouse, parent, worker, or friend—or at least not in the way she used to imagine. Betty comes to understand that her life has changed entirely and forever.

Psychological aspects. With the help and encouragement of her new MS friends and her team of the nurse practitioner and the social worker, she explores and expresses the grief she feels for the loss of her old self and she mourns the end of that life. Betty comes to wrestle with the reality that she "can't go home again."

Betty wonders, "Who am I?" "What good am I?" "Why did this happen to me?" "Why should I live?" "Is there any value to my life?" She goes through a terribly painful period in which she struggles to locate a meaning for her existence. Betty is very vulnerable at this time. She could become even more lost because of her own very considerable social withdrawal. She could fall victim to cynical and predatory providers. She could give way to despair and attempt to kill herself.

But Betty is fortunate. Her new friends and the nurse practitioner help Betty navigate the difficult course between necessary grieving for her past self and falling into severe clinical depression. Betty learns not to reject her new suffering self, but to have compassion instead. This isn't an easy task. She's constantly receiving messages from people in her society telling her that if she stays the way she is, if she remains ill, then they no longer want her among them.

To move forward from grief and mourning, Betty has to discover meaning for what has happened to her and find out what she can be in the future. She has to engage in philosophical or spiritual thinking in order to come to a new place. Betty begins by learning to respect the person she really is right now.

As is typically the case, Betty does this through a creative act. She decides to write a journal describing her experiences. Other people she knows have chosen things as various as taking up cooking, becoming MS advocates, or even remaking their wardrobe and hair style. One friend actually made a movie.

To accomplish her purpose, Betty draws heavily on the help and the faith of her care providers. She also draws extensively on a variety of wisdom traditions. Betty's not religious in the traditional sense. In fact, she regards herself as an atheist. But since she's consciously begun thinking about the basic issues of life and meaning, she's discovered aspects of Buddhism and Celtic philosophy that speak directly to her. In addition, Betty begins to read stories by other people with chronic illnesses. She discovers how these individuals have dealt with their disabilities, some of which are static, or unchanging (blindness, paraplegia), and some of which are dynamic, or changing, like hers. She becomes absorbed in accounts by survivors of all sorts—of disaster and imprisonment, as well as of illness. Guided by her social worker and by the inspiration of the heroic lives she's read about, Betty rewrites her own story in a positive way. She sees that she has a future. In the process of composing her narrative, Betty recreates herself and finds meaning in her experience.

Social and work aspects. Betty's positive psychological evolution during phase three doesn't occur in a benignly static social environment. In fact, Betty endures a considerable blow when she and Bob agree that they must divorce. At first Betty worries terribly about how she will manage. She still has a job at the bank, but she's always been on Bob's health plan. As part of the divorce settlement, he agrees to keep her and the children covered. As time passes, Bob demonstrates that he'll continue to meet his financial obligations to her and the children. He's also good about having the children regularly. This gives Betty needed quiet time and reduces her fears that the divorce will cause harmful distance between the children and their father.

Encouraged by one of her MS friends, Betty explicitly asks Lisa and Michael for help at home. She's surprised to find that Lisa responds enthusiastically, especially to cooking. Michael's good about drying dishes and putting in the laundry if he's reminded, but recently he's begun complaining about living with "a bunch of women." Betty couldn't have let him go two years ago, but now she's planning to let him spend his next school year with his father.

At the bank, Betty feels competent to deal with her present job require-ments. Toward the end of phase two, Betty's social worker came to the bank to discuss with Betty's supervisor how Betty could use her time and efforts most effectively and efficiently. With the supervisor's help, the social worker also organized a short meeting with Betty's co-workers. She informed them about MS, how it was affecting Betty, and answered their questions. As time has gone by since, Betty's co-workers have gotten so used to her condition that they have more or less forgotten it. Betty knows, however, that her job security depends almost entirely on her supervisor, so she's begun investi-gating other part-time work she might do, perhaps at home. The nurse-practitioner has also reminded Betty that she is eligible for disability if she is unable to work and Betty has been discussing this option with her social worker. She has also been inquiring among her MS friends about their experi-ences with disability.

In public Betty now refuses to pretend or to keep silent about her MS. When people react badly or seek to label or stigmatize her, she confronts them about their bias. She has been surprised at how empowered such behav-ior makes her feel. She has even thought about becoming formally involved in advocacy work. With the end of her marriage and the inevitable loss of some old friends and acquaintances, Betty has been forced to consider new roles and to seek new friends. She is amazed to find how positive this experi-ence is for her, and how much she likes her new self.

As Betty freely acknowledges, it would have been very hard for her to go through this time without the devoted and informed help of the nurse practitioner, the social worker, and her chronically ill friends who are strug-gling on the same journey that Betty is. She also includes as important mem-bers of her health-care team and support network those healthy people she has come to know who listen thoughtfully to what she says and make the effort to understand her situation. For most chronically ill patients, it takes experienced and devoted clinicians to guide them out of the potentially end-less loop of phase one and two and through the necessary developmental experiences of phase three.

Phase Four

Physical aspect. As in phase three, Betty may physically experience con-tinuous plateau, improved well-being, or relapse. But by now Betty recog-nizes the cyclic nature of her chronic disease and no longer sees relapse as a failure. Instead, she understands it as another cycle that she must once again integrate. She now realizes that this state of understanding and integration constitutes her recovery.

Psychological aspect. Betty has united the salvageable aspects of her pre-crisis self with her newly claimed and respected self. She maintains this achievement through a daily commitment to allow her suffering, to meet it with compassion, and to treat it with respect. This does not mean that life has become easy for Betty. Sometimes she cannot climb stairs at all. Sometimes she is so debilitated that she must use a wheelchair, which she hates. She can still become mentally confused, especially if she does too much. And she must daily perform small acts of bravery in the face of stigmatization, rejection, and even her own pain. But she stands with herself; she is conscious of her suffering, and this keeps her suffering from becoming neurotic. She has created a new "personal best," a new self-ideal to maintain.

Betty is also continuing to pursue philosophical and spiritual growth. She finds that a constant, active, conscious consideration of meaning and purpose enriches her life and places her experiences, both positive and negative, in a context larger than herself.

Social and work aspects. Betty continues to nurture the new friendships she began establishing in phase three. She has also managed to reintegrate some of her formerly alienated family and friends. Her frankness about her condition and her refusal to accept derogatory estimations make it perfectly clear to people who she is now. Some admire her for it and see the truth of her self-assessment.

Betty is about to change her job. While she worked at the bank and when she was at home sick, she became quite adept with computers, so she has decided to take a position running an MS Web site and chatroom. Although Bob has remarried—an event that threw Betty into emotional crisis—he is quite intrigued with her new job and enjoys discussing it with her. Relations between the two are better than they have been for a long time.

One of Betty's MS friends remarried recently. This gives Betty hope, and she's met a man she likes very much in a writing class. Because of his encouragement, she sent part of her journal to an MS newsletter, and the editors have asked whether she might like to contribute another piece.

Betty knows that crises and disasters happen all the time in life. She worries a lot about her children. A friend of Michael's was just arrested for stealing a car. She thinks that Lisa may have had a pregnancy scare. One of her MS friends took a terrible turn for the worse and will probably not survive. This scares Betty terribly, for she knows the same could happen to her. But Betty is learning to separate those things she can control from those she can't. While it's a continuous effort, she tries to exert herself with regard to the things she can affect and to endure with grace those she can't.

Chronically ill individuals in phase four have only occasional need for clinical help. If a serious blow knocks them back into phase one, they may turn again to a helpful clinician to speed the process of integrating the experience into their lives. And frequently they keep in touch out of friendship. But for the most part they can manage living with their chronic illness by themselves.

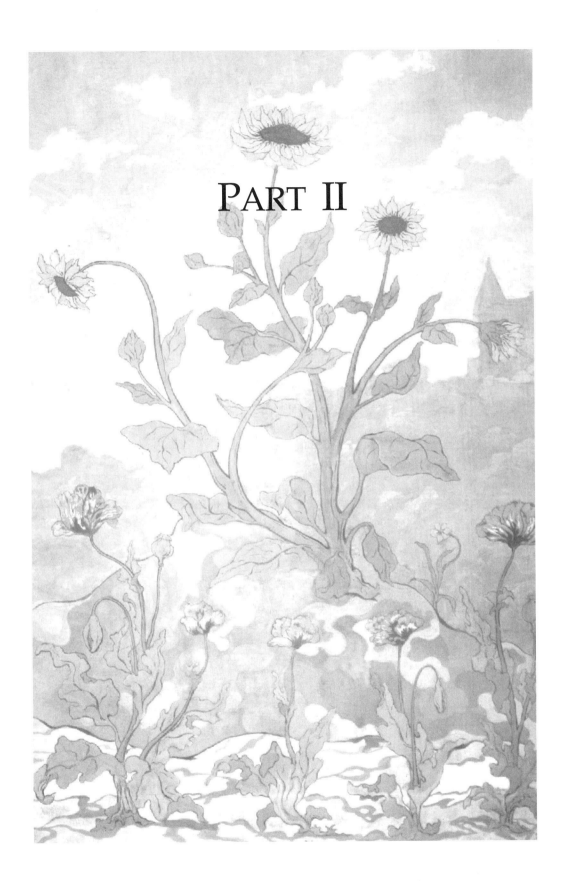

PART II

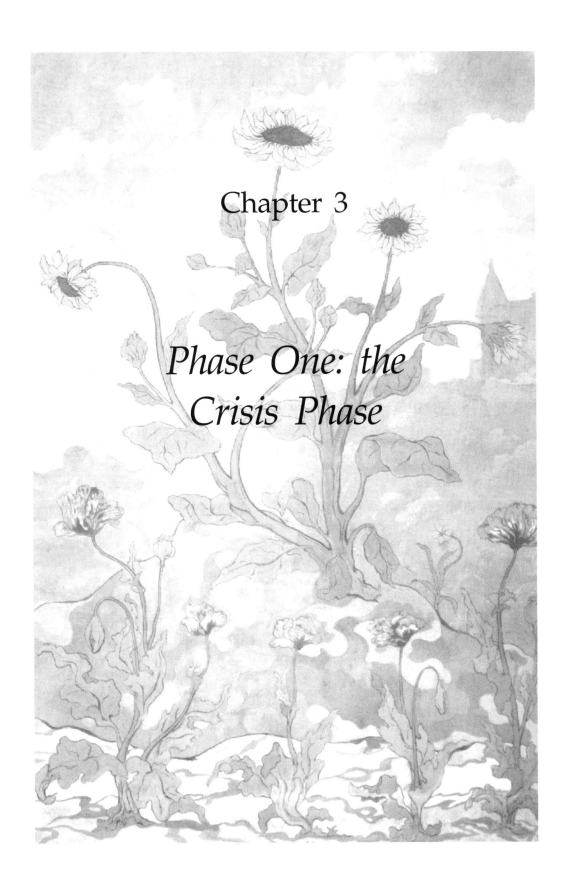

Chapter 3

Phase One: the Crisis Phase

Before I talk with you specifically about what you need to do when you're in phase one, I want to share with you my overall approach. In each phase I'm going to give you a **strategy**. This strategy is the broad, overall way you're going to achieve the goal of each phase. Next, I'll list a variety of **tactics** to help you accomplish the strategy, and I'll teach you the **skills** you'll need to carry out the tactics. Finally, I'll introduce some **coping and comfort** activities that will help you live a little more satisfactorily as you navigate through the phase.

I also want to remind you that you'll want to make several copies of the blank exercises in the next chapters. It helps to have several copies, just in case you want to change what you've written. Also, you'll be completing some of these exercises several times.

Crisis

You feel urgency. The period of crisis is an extremely disorienting time. With the onset of your illness, your world can be turned completely upside down. You may feel, like Betty did, that you absolutely must find out what is happening to you—what is going wrong. And you very likely feel that you have to find this out just as soon as possible.

Help can come only from outside. Probably you also feel that you can't do anything about your situation yourself. You've already tried. It's going to take other people—specialists, experts, doctors—to help you. They're the only ones who can figure out what's wrong and how to treat and cure you.

You think you're to blame. Perhaps you think that you have some rare condition, but even if you think your problem may be commonplace, you may feel that you're to blame. You can feel you brought this all on yourself and that you're making your family suffer, too. If you truly had done things differently, you might not be sick now. Perhaps, if you were a better person, you wouldn't be punished this way.

You have upsetting thoughts. You may find yourself thinking very upsetting thoughts over and over again. You just can't seem to get them out of your head. You may think all the time about your symptoms or pain and how you can't stand the way things are. You may think sometimes about how you'd be better off dead. These thoughts, combined with all the other strange things that are happening to you, make you fearful. You wonder if you're going crazy. Your negative thoughts distract you from your work or keep you from sleep.

You're not acting like yourself. Maybe you've found yourself starting to behave in ways that aren't like you at all. The harder you keep struggling to perform your usual roles and jobs, the more difficult it becomes and the more you feel like you're ripping apart at the seams. Betty, you remember, began crying in public places. This was something that she had never done before, even when she had good reasons to cry. Yet here she was in a meeting at work or looking at packages of chicken in the supermarket with tears streaming down her face. All the physical changes she was experiencing, together with all the losses these changes were causing, were overwhelming her. Of course, crying in public didn't make Betty feel better. Instead, it made everything even worse, including how Betty felt about herself. If you've found yourself behaving in ways that just aren't like you, maybe you're as overwhelmed as Betty was. In addition, you're probably scared—not just because you're having uncomfortable, perhaps painful physical symptoms, but also because you're confused and not sure which way to turn.

This is what it feels like to be in crisis.

Strategy: Going into the Bunker

Goal. The goal in phase one is to contain the crisis. I call this strategy "going into the bunker," meaning that you're going to get into a manageable, secure place where you'll be safe while you figure out what to do next.

The strategy for containing the crisis includes three key components. One is for the physical you, who's feeling pain or exhaustion and debilitation. The next is for the "inside" you, who can be feeling fear, confusion, grief, anger, and frustration. And the last helps you relate more successfully to the people around you in your family, your community, and your workplace.

Staying safe physically. First, you need a safety plan for dealing with the emotional and physical earthquake that comes with illness onset. Physical pain, mental changes, mood swings, physical limitations, not to mention emotional frustration, denial, and grief put you at risk for problems in addition to those you already have. It's essential to make sure that you're safe while you're going through the shock of your disease onset. You need to get yourself into a safe, earthquake-proof bunker.

Hanging on psychologically. You also need to learn how to hang on mentally and emotionally while you're battered around by the changes and suffering you're experiencing.

Working with others. Finally, you need to understand how the people around you are reacting to your illness. You must also learn how to help counteract the bad effects their negative behavior can have on you and utilize the support available to you.

Tactics and Skills

Staying Safe Physically

See Your Doctor

In this book, I've assumed up to this point that a trained and licensed medical professional has already diagnosed you as having a chronic illness or syndrome. However, if you've been having symptoms, but have *not* yet seen a doctor, you should make an appointment. You need to begin the process of discovering what's going on with your body from a medical perspective. Some things need to be ruled out right away. It's also quite possible that you have an acute condition that can be treated in a fairly straightforward way. And if you don't have an easily treated illness, you need to begin the process of pursuing a diagnosis and getting your physical symptoms monitored under a physician's care.

Get a Doctor You Like and Trust

If you don't like the physician you're currently seeing, you should find one you do like. This person should be a qualified professional who listens to you carefully and treats you with respect. If you need to find a physician, skip ahead to chapter 7. It gives some specific steps so you can find the right doctor for you.

Your Health-Care Team

Just like everybody else with a chronic illness, you need a health-care team to help you and your family manage the illness experience. What team members you get will vary depending on your specific illness, but here are some basics to consider.

Your health-care team will perform certain basic functions. They will determine what specific treatment protocols are necessary at each phase of your illness, and one or two of them will oversee and coordinate all aspects of your health care. Given how our health-care system is currently structured, your health-care players may not be used to assuming this oversight responsibility. They can, however, be asked to take on that role, and they'll be more inclined to accept when they see that you'll share the job with them.

Primary-care physician. First of all, you must definitely have a primary-care physician. This doctor acts as your gatekeeper to the other specialists you may require. This person also will help to advocate for you with your HMO regarding specific services.

Primary-care manager. In reality, the doctor's office staff will be performing many of the services you need, so it's important to identify the person in your doctor's office who's going to act as your primary-care manager. The doctor usually assesses your symptoms and decides what physical treatment steps you should take. But he or she may also delegate authority to a physician's assistant in the office or, more frequently, to a nurse practitioner. While the primary-care physician oversees the work of these individuals, your care manager will more often have the time necessary to coordinate and manage cases of chronic illness.

Social worker or psychologist. The doctor's office may refer you to a social worker, an occupational therapist, or a psychologist so that you and your family can get the help you need in managing all the changes the illness experience has caused in your life. If you haven't been referred to such people, you should ask your doctor's office for a referral. These professionals work specifically in areas of your life that are unaddressed by physical medicine. For many people with chronic illnesses, the kinds of problems these professionals help solve are often ultimately more distressing than the actual illness itself. Because a number of different specialists may be helpful in similar ways, I'm going to refer to this person from now on as your *counselor*. Remember, your counselor may be a social worker, a psychologist, or some other licensed professional.

Team leader. The doctor or nurse practitioner and the counselor or psychologist are the two key players on your health-care team. One of them shares a leading role. The two of you will make sure to keep information flowing among all the team members. Depending on your particular needs, any team member may recommend that you add other team players. For example, you may be having sleep difficulties. This may not come to light until a discussion you and your partner or spouse have with the counselor. It's frequently a partner who recognizes that the patient is not sleeping well. At that point the counselor will contact your physical-care manager and together they'll arrange for referral to a sleep specialist. Or your doctor may notice that you are becoming increasingly scared about your new chronic illness and its disabilities. This is hardly unusual. Most people experience all these changes as a serious crisis. The doctor may want to prescribe medication that will help to manage your emotional symptoms, but first he or she may also contact your counselor to discuss what kinds of steps you and your family might take instead of medication or in addition to it.

Changes on the team. As you move through the chronic illness phases, your health-care team will most likely change. For example, if you have MS, it may be appropriate for you to be evaluated by a neurologist in phase one. If you have fibromyalgia, it may be appropriate for you to see a rheumatologist. You may need the help of an occupational therapist as you attempt to restructure your basic activities of daily living. In phase two it's quite likely that you would benefit from an evaluation by a physical or occupational therapist. These additional or auxiliary health-care providers assess your situation and make recommendations to you and your team-management leader so that you can make needed treatment decisions.

Keeping the team informed. You and all of your clinical team players need to be kept informed about changes in your condition or alterations in your physical protocols or medications. Usually the team leader works closely with your primary physician. But anyone on the team, particularly the team leader, should question any plans or protocols that seem to contradict other protocols or medications. The team leader also should look into any negative side effects that the protocols or medications create. This is why you want to be completely candid with your team leader. Your counselor needs to know and understand what medical findings have been made and when additional protocols have been ordered. Your primary-care physician and nurse practitioner need to know and understand the assessments that the counselor has made and the kinds of interventions they are planning.

Prior medical history. Everybody on your team, including you, needs to understand your prior medical history and any problems in that history that can affect your chronic illness. For instance, if you tell your counselor that you have poor toleration of certain medications, the counselor may then want to recommend a medication review for you. Similarly, it's important for your doctor to learn what you've been telling your counselor, or perhaps what your spouse has been telling your counselor. For example, you may have told your counselor that every time you come home from your new exercise program your symptoms are worse, in which case your exercise regimen may be adjusted.

Physical Health-Care Goals

It's very important to follow your health-care protocols, since they can improve your quality of life. Because this compliance is so important, you need to set up some physical health-care goals. These may include setting up a system to ensure that you take your medications at the right times of day every day. Or you may set specific daily goals about your eating habits. Some people with chronic illnesses don't tolerate wheat very well. They can't comfortably digest ordinary pastas, breads, or other baked products. They need help first in selecting alternative foods that they like and then in sticking to their new diet. Perhaps a sleep disorder is part of your clinical picture. In that case you'll need help setting up specific behavioral goals that address your sleep habits. To make sure that you know all the tasks you need to account for, complete Exercise 1, "List of Health-Care Tasks."

In Exercise 1, you want to note your medications and when you take them. You need to consider any special exercises you must perform regularly to keep the mobility you still have. You may also have special care tasks that may be as minor as remembering to use artificial tears or as major as regularly cleansing an ostomy. In phase 1 many people have a variety of diagnostic tests to schedule. You should note these on your list and insert the dates of the tests when you have made appointments for them. In the section on diet you'll want to itemize foods that you should include in your diet and foods you should avoid. If foods you should avoid include a major food component such as wheat, make a list of possible substitutes. Finally, if you have sleep issues, you should note the clinical recommendations for improving your sleep habits.

Exercise 1
List of Health-Care Tasks

Medications

Name	Times per day	Hours to take

Physical Regimes
Daily exercises

Exercise and how done	Number of times	When in day

Special cleaning/care

Activity	Number of times	Supplies needed

Tests

Tests ordered	Date scheduled	Requirements

Diet

Foods required _____

_____

_____

Foods to avoid _____

_____

_____

Possible substitutes _____

_____

_____

Sleep

Special requirements _____

_____

_____

Emergency List

You also need to make an emergency list. This list is different for different people because it depends on your particular problems. For example, if you are taking drugs that impair your ability to drive, you need to have a list of people or organizations you can call if you need to be taken somewhere. Or you may need to make sure that you have someone who can buy groceries for you at those times when you can't get out shopping yourself. Perhaps your cognitive difficulties make it difficult for you to pay your bills, so you need to set up automatic bill-paying or find a service to do your bills. Perhaps your physical debilitation is such that you sometimes need help with personal hygiene activities like bathing, washing your hair, or doing your laundry. In this case you may need help from a friend or perhaps a home-health aide. Exercise 2, "Emergency List," helps you create your personal emergency list. The section for medical emergencies should include the number to call if you have bad reactions to medications. Your medical emergency numbers should be parties who will answer twenty-four-hours a day.

Assessing Your Activity Threshold

In addition to assessing the medical aspects of your physical situation, you and your health-team leader need to figure out what your activity threshold is right now, while you are in crisis. This is very important. On the one hand, being in crisis reduces your physical, cognitive, and emotional ability to take on new tasks. At the same time, however, the changes brought on by the crisis almost always create more work for you, not less. In addition to everything else, you have medical appointments to meet and medical protocols to carry out. You need to discover how much you can do so that you won't always be trying to do too much and getting sicker because you do.

Categories of Activities

The activities in your life generally fall into four categories. The first are the activities of daily living (the ADLs). These include personal care, laundry, food purchasing, food preparation, house cleaning, car maintenance, bill paying, house repairs, and other things that keep the daily business of your life going. The second category includes activities that relate to your personal enrichment or fulfillment. Some people think of this group as including activities related to personal growth. For one person this may mean playing golf or taking bike rides, or camping, but activities can also include reading, attending musical concerts, going back to college, or attending religious services. The third category includes all activities related to your life as a social person. These range from the things you do for and with your family to interaction with friends and engagement in community activities. The fourth category includes all activities related to work or employment. Obviously, some activities overlap categories, and people may also argue about what category an activity fits into.

Exercise 2
Emergency List

Medical Emergencies

Person or Contact	Phone number

Physical Care Needs
(can be visiting nurse, home health aide, family member, or friend)

	Person or Contact	Phone number
Medications		
Laundry		
Bathing, hair, etc.		

Food

	Person or Contact	Phone number
Shopping		
Preparation		

Transportation

	Person or Contact	Phone number
Regular		
Occasional		

Financial

	Person or Contact	Phone number
Bill-paying		
Other (specify)		

As an example, let's look briefly at Caroline's experience. Caroline works full-time as a computer programmer. She also looks after most of her children's daily living needs. At first glance, taking care of her children might seem to be a social activity for Caroline because it's a family activity. But some people would argue that family activities are their emotional sharing and engagement activities. And some would say that washing the kids' clothes and fixing their school lunches are actually work activities, just like Caroline's programming job. As another example, some people would argue that their volunteer activity at a community center really fits into the personal fulfillment category, not the social category. For now, what you need to understand is that you perform many different kinds of activities, and that each of these activities falls into one of four large categories.

Your Physical Constitution

You may remember that back in your grandparents' day, people used to talk about a person's physical strength in terms of the individual's having a strong or weak constitution. They meant that some people seemed to be able to do huge amounts of work without getting tired, while others who were perfectly healthy seemed to tire more quickly. This notion of a person's constitution is still useful, especially when you're trying to figure out what you're capable of doing now, given your current situation.

Different constitutions. Not every healthy person has the same level of physical hardiness. In your pre-illness life you may have regularly gone rock climbing, hiking, or jogging. But a lot of people think that walking around the block is serious exercise. One parent of three small children will chase up and down stairs after them, do the laundry, make the meals, clean them up, get them into bed, and still have energy left over after the kids are asleep. Another parent is winded getting one squirmy kid dressed in the morning.

Your constitution is part of who you are. It's important to find out what your constitution was like before you became ill, compared with what you're like now. Your constitution will have been a major part of your personal identity. And what your constitution used to be shapes your expectations now about how much you should be able to do every day, whether you're able to or not.

If you have been sick your entire life, or most of your adult life, it is important for you to think about what your constitution is like when you're feeling good. You'll probably have to use your imagination. When things are going well, do you feel energetic and eager to do a lot of different things? Or, on your good days, do you feel that you can do some things but not a lot? It's important for you to have a notion of your benchmark constitution because you'll need it to help set up levels of activity that are appropriate for you.

In order to get a sense of where you are now compared to where you used to be, you're going to fill out Exercise 3, "Activity Analysis." First, you need to think back and try to recreate what you did on a typical day before you got sick. The first page captures what you typically did daily, and the second page calls for information about how much energy you expended on special occasions. Since you're trying to remember how you used to be, you'll be estimating your benchmark constitution. Try to make your estimate as accurate as possible so it will to be useful to you later. Don't exaggerate how much you did and don't minimize it.

Now, to capture your present condition, you need to make seven copies of the first page of the exercise. You're going to fill these out for each day of one week. Make sure to write the day and date at the top of each sheet so that you don't get confused about which days you've done. On the second page of Exercise 3, you're going to list the activities and time you now spend on special occasions and vacations.

These nontypical activities may have played a significant role in your life, so it is important to try to capture how much time you used to spend doing them and how much time you spend on them now. On vacations, for example, some families go away to the mountains or the seashore and "rough it" for a couple of weeks. If you're the person responsible for cooking and washing clothes, you may expend far more effort on "vacation" than you do when you're at home.

Try to be realistic, about both the past and your current state. Typically, people with chronic illnesses actually accomplish a lot less than they want to accomplish. This has nothing to do with whether you're a competitive, hard-driving, accomplishment-oriented personality. It happens because your chronic illness makes it impossible for you to do all the things that you used to do before you got sick. At the same time, some people who are sick often romanticize the past and think they did more than they really did because now they can do so little.

Activities of Daily Living

The activities of daily living—doing your own cooking, cleaning, laundry, caring for yourself personally—are probably the most important activities that you do every day. In today's world, people tend to discount ADLs because nearly everyone has to do them. Some people even have to accomplish most of the ADLs for other people, like their children or a partner, as well as their own. Actually, other people's ADLs are work activities for the people who carry them out. But if these people stop doing them, someone else has to take up the slack. There are also some who hire people to carry out many of their ADLs. But if these people can't work when they get sick and no longer have the income to pay others, they suddenly face the prospect of having to do their ADLs themselves. Most people also forget how much effort ADLs actually take. You know that none of them happens by itself automatically, and yet you tend to think these aren't jobs at all. You probably don't regard cleaning your apartment as equal to conducting a management meeting at work, but in reality it probably requires a lot more physical effort. Your ability to carry out daily activities is central to your ability to survive. But

Exercise 3
Activity Analysis

Day and Date _____

Daily activities

Time of day	List of activities	Total hrs/item
Morning activities (includes washing, dressing, bed-making, breakfast, making lunches, getting kids ready, walking pets, etc.)		
Morning at work/home (itemize typical activities, including weekend jobs and activities)		
Noon/lunch time (includes going out, doing errands, etc.)		
Afternoon at work/home		
Dinnertime (preparation, serving, cleanup)		
Evening		

Nontypical activity periods

	List occasions, number of days/activities involved	Total hours
Holidays		
Birthdays		
Other special occasions		
Vacations (note esp. strenuous physical activities)		

equally important, your ability to carry out ADLs is also central to your self-esteem.

Exercise 4, "Responsibilities, Expectations, and Desires," helps you capture important information about what you have to do and what you expect and want from your life. You will fill out three columns describing these three things. "Responsibilities" describe the minimum that you are required to do at work and at home because of your job description and your share in the family division of household responsibilities. "Expectations" captures the level of activity on the job and at home that makes you feel like you're carrying out your responsibilities well. "Desires" measures the ideal that you'd like to achieve in all your various activities and includes activities that you wish you could do but do not have the time, energy, or resources to carry out. This last might include quitting full-time work so you can take up pottery-making or go windsurfing. Or it might mean returning to college to get training for a different, more desirable kind of career.

Exercise 4
Responsibilities, Expectations, and Desires

Responsibilities	Expectations	Desires
At home:	At home:	
At work:	At work:	

Exercise 5, "Tracking Daily Symptoms," provides you with the final vital area of information that you'll need to help you begin to restructure your activities. You will fill out Exercise 5 each day for a week. First, however, you need to revise the list of symptoms in the left-hand column to fit your condition. In general, however, your symptom list will probably include fatigue, pain, cognitive problems, anxiety, and depression.

Before you fill out the first sheet, you also need to establish a scale for the severity of your symptoms. Assign numbers, from 1 to 5, to grade your pain. Number 1 is the best, and 5 is the worst. Do not count as 1 that wonderful day when you had no troubles at all. Your 1 should be the best *average* sort of day. Similarly, 5 does not mean unbearable pain or total cognitive confusion, but the worst of a bad *average* day. Write your pain scale on the back of your first day's Exercise 5 to help you remember.

At the top of each day's sheet for Exercise 5, write in the day and date and, if you have menstrual cycles, what day in your cycle it is.

Next, check "Yes" or "No" as to whether you have "resting symptoms." Resting symptoms are symptoms you have when you're relaxed, lying down, and not expending any effort at all.

Finally, in the upper section of Exercise 5, evaluate your previous night's sleep. Your evaluation should include time—starting when you actually put your head on the pillow until you finally got up for the following day. You should note how long it took you to fall asleep and how many times you awoke during the night. If you woke during the night, record how long it took you to get back to sleep again. Remember to include any night sweats or chills and any light, dream-laden sleeping. If you've got to get up frequently at night to urinate, note that as well.

On the lower part of Exercise 5 you'll track your actual daily symptoms by assigning a number for each part of the day to each symptom. Make the times of day fit your actual day. Your morning, for example, may begin at 6 A.M. or it may begin at 11 A.M. Roughly speaking, you want to think of "morning" as being the time from when you get up until you need your midday meal. "Afternoon" is the time from your midday meal until your meal at the end of the day, and "evening" is that time after your final meal of the day.

New Activity Boundaries

As you review the results of Exercises 3, 4, and 5, you should begin to see very specifically how you're using up your available energy and what effect it's having on you. After examining these results, you'll have the information you need to begin establishing your new activity boundaries. For example, maybe you used to go to a weight and fitness program three times a week before the onset of your illness, and you'd like to continue. Or perhaps your doctor suggested that you join an aerobics class because the doctor thinks that this will give you a desirable amount of regulated physical activity. You see, from examining your lists, that doing grocery shopping, carting

Exercise 5
Tracking Daily Symptoms

Day and date: _____   Date in menstrual cycle (if appropriate): _____

Resting symptoms   ☐ Yes   ☐ No

Evaluation of previous night's sleep _____

_____

_____

Symptoms	Morning	Afternoon	Evening
Fatigue			
Cognitive			
Headache			
Sore throat			
Body ache			
GI problems			
Anxiety			
Depression			

in the bundles, and putting everything away is just about all the physical exercise you can handle right now. Much as you'd like to exercise the standard three times a week, perhaps for now you can go only once a week. Later, when you're in better health, you may be able to increase the frequency of your formal exercise. If your activity exercises reveal that you're severely compromised physically, your new physical boundaries may consist solely of getting out of bed, dressing in your street clothes, and eating with your family.

Trading off activities or rearranging them. One way to gain maximum use of your available energy is learning how to trade off activities. On a day when you shop for groceries, for example, you won't wash your hair, prepare any meals, or pick up the children from daycare. If you're still able to work, you may find you use your limited energy more effectively by shaving and showering in the evening, rather than using up valuable morning energy on such tasks. You may find it helpful to set up your breakfast things the night before and to lay out the clothes you plan to wear the following day. Your goal here is to reduce the number of "keystrokes" in your life. You may find that your counselor or an occupational therapist can be very helpful to you in these efforts.

Revising your expectations. By comparing Exercise 4 to Exercises 3 and 5, you can also see how much your expectations, desires, and probably your responsibilities exceed what you're capable of doing at the present time. You want to begin thinking about ways to revise your personal norms to fit with your current physical state. Revision of personal norms is a very complex activity and almost always requires help. Your counselor is an excellent person to work with. A little further along in the book we'll talk about choosing an activity gatekeeper. This person can also be very helpful as you try to revise your personal norms.

Exercise 6, "Paring Down Activities," suggests some slightly humorous but necessary activities to help teach you how to reduce the demands you make on yourself. Even when you're not feeling your best you'll want to make your best effort sometimes, but it helps not to expend so much energy all the time. Try to do one activity in each section of Exercise 6 one or two times weekly. You might like to try inventing some paring-down activities of your own, as well as those in the exercise.

Small steps for a bit of control. It's probably already occurred to you that your life is going to require complex activity restructuring. But now, in phase one, all you're trying to do is create a system that works for you so that you can carry out the basic activities of living. Even if you're still going to work, you want to focus almost entirely during this crisis phase on restructuring your ADLs. If you can set up a workable system for them, you'll begin to feel a small degree of control returning to your life. This bit of control is going to help you get through the crisis.

Exercise 6
Paring Down Activities

This is a kind of game. Try doing any of these suggestions (or your own inventions along the same line) once or twice a week.

At home

1. When you wash the dishes, leave two items unwashed in the sink.

2. Do not sort or open the mail when you come home. Put it on your desk until after you take a rest.

3. See how disheveled (some may say relaxed) you can allow yourself to look at home in the evening or on Saturday morning. Can you not comb your hair? Wear comfortable sloppy old clothes? Not wear a bra? Not wear anything with a belt?

At Work

1. Do not read anything in your inbox that doesn't require immediate attention.

2. Purposely do not do one non-urgent task.

3. Do not return non-urgent phone calls immediately.

4. Do not refile folders on your desk at the end of the day.

With Friends

1. Do not try to keep the conversation rolling. Let others do the work.

2. Try being the strong, silent type.

3. See how long you can go on in a conversation using only one-syllable responses. (Be sure to tell your friend that you're going to give this activity a try ahead of time.)

4. When talking, lower your voice and speak more slowly.

Trying to "Pass"

If you're like most people with a chronic illness, you don't have a really good sense of your new physical, psychological, or social boundaries or limitations. Most chronically ill people try very hard to continue being the person they always used to be in the outside world. Like them, you're probably trying to act as though you're "healthy" and "normal." If your condition gives you some cognitive difficulties, it's even harder to pass, because if people see that you're having trouble thinking or figuring things out, you're afraid they'll think you're crazy or look foolish. In all three aspects of your life— your physical life, your psychological or emotional life, and your social and work life—you're almost surely trying to do everything that you used to do and, given your new medical protocols, maybe even more. Trying to pass, however, often leads to a collapse.

Learning from the Experience of Collapse

If you've overdone things and had the misfortune to suffer a distinct worsening of your condition as a consequence, it would be nice to think that you could at least learn from the experience. But most people don't. You don't want to believe that you're sick or disabled. You also probably believe that you wouldn't have had that collapse if you had just tried harder. You probably think you didn't make the necessary effort. When people are in crisis, they usually blame themselves when things go wrong rather than blame their illnesses.

Making a New Daily Schedule

In Exercise 7, "Daily Schedule," you're going to try to create a reasonable weekly schedule for your life as you're living it right now. What activities you can accomplish will change in the future, so your daily schedule will also change. But right now you're almost certainly doing too much. You've got to cut back in a way that allows you to meet your responsibilities without exhausting yourself. If you can't meet your responsibilities even when you cut back, then you need to talk with your health-care team leader about finding the help you need to survive.

Including all activity categories. As you fill out Exercise 7, you want to make sure that you include a detailed list of activities. You want to make sure, for example, that you've included all your ADLs—including washing yourself, brushing your teeth, combing your hair, and so on. You can certainly perform some of them less frequently, and you may need to ask for help from others to perform some of them. If you're still working, you need to include all your required job activities and how you get to and from work. If you are living with a partner or family, you need to think about how you've rearranged your roles and responsibilities. We'll talk more about this in the next section. You need to include some time with friends, even though you may visit with them mostly by phone or e-mail. And finally—even though you're cutting way down on all your activities—*you need to include*

Exercise 7
Daily Schedule

	Early A.M.	Morning at work/home	Lunchtime	Afternoon at work/home	Dinner prep/cleanup	Evening
Monday						
Tuesday						
Wednesday						
Thursday						
Friday						
Saturday						
Sunday						

some time for activities of personal fulfillment. In the crisis phase, you should try to make these quiet, placid activities, because you're trying to reduce energy expenditure until you get a better handle on your chronic illness. Nonetheless, it is important to think about all four general categories of activity and to try to include some things from each category.

If you don't have enough space for all your activities on Exercise 7, make your own schedule on separate sheets of paper. Using Exercise 7 as a guide, list the days of the week on the left side of your paper and list the activity headings along the top. Allow plenty of room to list *all* of your activities.

Getting an Activity Gatekeeper

One way to help yourself control your expenditure of energy is by finding an activity gatekeeper. This person is usually either your counselor or a particularly close friend rather than your partner or a family member. Your activity gatekeeper is someone you like and trust, someone who can tell you things you don't want to hear. You tell this person about your situation and how you've got to be careful about how much you do. You ask him or her to keep track of you and to tell you when they think you're doing too much. Most of us don't see things about ourselves that are obvious to our good friends. Your activity gatekeeper may be able to help you avoid a relapse by warning you that you're exhausting yourself. During the crisis phase, especially while you're creating a new daily schedule, you'll want to consult with your gatekeeper regularly. Your gatekeeper may recognize that your plan itself still contains too many activities each day, or may observe when you get together that you haven't reduced your activities enough because you're still exhausting yourself.

Hanging On Psychologically

Changes in Time

One of the things that probably stands out in your life now is how much your experience of time changed when you got sick. This is a very common experience. Scientists have discovered that high stress or trauma releases chemicals in the brain that slow people's perception of time. The experience of time is significant in all four phases, but during the crisis phase, time changes dramatically. It's as if time has stopped for you, and you're trapped in a time warp. It can seem like the rest of the world is still moving forward—in fact, is moving forward at an ever-increasing speed—and you feel like you're being left behind. Some people talk about this experience as being like B.C. and A.D. in the time schemes of their personal histories. Because of the urgency you may also be experiencing in this crisis phase, your experience of time can make you feel like you're being held captive. Your thoughts, your pain, and your fear—all perfectly typical of this phase—are part of what keeps you confined. We'll come back to this experience of time as we move through the phases. For now, what's important is that you understand how uncomfortable your experience of time can be during the crisis phase and how typical it is of everyone. It's not happening only to you.

Your Public Self and Your Private Self

Everyone has a public self, the "face" and behavior we present to the world. We also have a private self, those parts that we share only with people who are very close to us. With your spouse or partner, for example, you may talk baby talk. Or you may talk out loud to yourself when you're alone. In private you may cry over minor matters. This behavior comes from your private self and expresses very private feelings. Your public self tends to be more "grown up." It censors the feelings of your private self so that you don't express them in public unless they are "appropriate."

But once you've entered the crisis phase, you may be shocked to find that you're sometimes behaving in an unexpected and embarrassing way in public. Perhaps you've burst into tears at the supermarket, or felt overwhelmed and then heard yourself complaining out loud about how much you have to do at home and at work. You may even speak differently from usual. Your voice may seem young, even childish. You may find that you're carrying yourself differently. You may feel awkward, unsure, even insecure, as you try to explain something to someone or ask for something that you need. Basically, depending on the intensity of the crisis that you're going through, you may not be able to maintain your public self all the time. It's not at all unusual for your private self, with its personal feelings and behavior, to break through into social and work situations.

This sudden emotional shift is normal in the crisis phase, regardless of who you are or how emotionally hardy you were prior to your illness. For most people, this intrusion of the private self is a way of working through a very difficult time. You can think of it as you becoming your most primitive self—as though you were a little kid again. Once you learn new coping skills, you'll probably find that the balance returns between your private self and your public self.

Such a big change in emotion and personality can be frightening, however, both to you and to the people around you. This is a difficulty you don't have to work out by yourself. It is something that the counselor on your health-care team can help you with. Often this person is also your team leader, which is really convenient. It's very important that you share these kinds of emotional experiences with your team.

If you or your family has had a history of emotional difficulties or mental illness, then your team leader needs to factor this information into the plans for helping you. It's important to remember, however, that people who've never had any difficulties at all emotionally nearly always experience some degree of imbalance between their public and private selves. It comes in response to the mounting problems of your illness.

Since these feelings and behaviors seem to come out of nowhere—you may not even realize what's happening to you—you can feel ashamed and embarrassed by yourself. Increasingly you may be afraid you're crazy or dying from some as yet undiagnosed disease. Your loss of ego—of your old self—can be very substantial.

Emotional Passing

Despite all these changes, you're probably still trying to pass for emotionally normal, just as you're probably trying to pass for physically normal. This is very typical behavior in phase one. Most people in the crisis phase have very little sense of their new emotional abilities and boundaries. People tend to fall into one of two general groups: conscious passers and unconscious passers. Unconscious passers sincerely deny that their illness has caused them any loss or change in functioning. They may acknowledge that they occasionally have emotional outbursts or sometimes experience confusion, but they simply don't believe or perceive that such events will happen to them as a regular thing. People who pass consciously know they've got a problem, but they don't want anyone else to see it. Like the unconscious passers, they have little accurate sense of their emotional abilities and boundaries, but they attempt to keep close track of how they're acting and try to make it look as normal as possible. If they've got problems figuring out a mathematical problem at work, for example, they won't ask for help. Instead, they'll sneak the problem home and struggle to figure it out there where no one will see how much time they're taking. If they do ask for help, they pretend it's for another reason. It's not that they don't understand the problem, but that they don't have their glasses with them or some other excuse. Regardless of whether you're a conscious or unconscious passer, passing largely results from your sense of shame. Emotional passing is, however, a way to cope. Once you've contained your crisis and entered phase two, you'll learn how to use emotional passing behavior consciously and constructively for personal protection and for rehabilitative purposes.

Changes Your Friends Observe

Almost inevitably you're less active and less lively than you used to be before you became ill. You probably have increasing difficulty interacting with other people at all. At the very least, *how* you interact changes. You simply can't expend the effort you used to, so you may speak less, talk in a lower voice, gesture less. Your family, friends, and co-workers notice this and may comment on how you've changed, even though they may not know you're ill. *It's okay for you to change*. Actually, you've got to, because you must adapt to your new circumstances. But it's often difficult for you not to be alarmed when people comment on the difficult changes you're going through. In the long run, some of the changes may be ones you want to keep even when your circumstances change. Many chronically ill people find that the ways they learned to behave when they had to change have made them more patient and more reflective. They don't care to change back to how they used to be even though they regain greater levels of energy.

Equal, Supportive Clinical Relationships

Given all the experiences you're having, it's important for you to have a good relationship with your team leader and with your counselor. It's important that you feel that you and your clinician are comrades traveling on this journey together. You'll need to have a gut sense that each of these people sees you as a partner, as someone who's just as human as she or he is. Your team leader has to see you as someone who's worthy of the same level of respect from the world at large that anyone else receives. Of course, you want these team members to be expert in matters that you don't understand, but that expertise should not permit them to act or behave as "better" or superior human beings, different from yourself.

Illness affirmation. This clinician must affirm your illness experience, especially since so many people around you do not. In fact, they're frequently discounting your experience completely. It's important for you to know that your clinician believes you and is sympathetic to what you're going through. How can you tell this about people? You'll know by their words, by how they look at you, and by their body language. Are they just listening, or do they really seem to hear and process what you need to tell them? You should feel that your clinician likes you and is truly concerned about your well-being. Your clinician shouldn't seem like someone just doing a job.

Trauma affirmation. Phase one is a time of crisis, and consequently it can be a time of trauma for you and the people around you. Trauma comes in many forms, not the least of which is the experience of being rejected by others because you're ill or disabled. It's important for you to understand that trauma frequently comes with illness. It's sometimes unavoidable. Using this book, you and your counselor need to examine the traumas that have occurred to you and those around you. You need to begin to grieve for the ways in which your illness has disrupted or even destroyed the life you once had. Your clinician should have the professional experience to help you begin to take control of your new reality, including the change that may have occurred in your sense of time, your urgency, your sense of self-blame, your emotional storms, and your need to pass for normal.

Loss, Grief, and Fear

Difficult as it is to think about loss, grief, and fear, it's essential work for you in phase one. Accounting for the losses your illness has brought to your life and beginning to grieve for them are some of the most important processes of phase one. Working on these issues with a counselor can make a huge difference. This clinician can help you identify losses that you find nearly impossible to confront. A counselor can help you understand what's your responsibility and what isn't. You can learn to grieve for things you couldn't help losing. Many people in phase one have endured terrible losses. Some are social, some are psychological, and some involve work. Maybe you feel like you can't be a partner at home the way you used to be, or the employee you used to be on the job. Maybe you're too tired to participate with your friends and family the way you used to. Maybe you're trying as hard as you can to keep up, but nevertheless you're failing all the time. Maybe you feel terribly isolated and alone because no one, not even the people closest to you, can grasp what you're going through even if they want to. Your social losses can be matched by inner losses. Maybe you look at yourself and don't recognize what you see because you're so different now. Small wonder that you may think you're crazy or dying or worse.

The Big Connection

It's time for you to learn the "big connection." This is the idea that illness creates trauma, loss, and grief and that this trauma, loss, and grief must be affirmed and then expressed deliberately. Otherwise, you'll find that your body will express them anyway at inconvenient times and in ineffective and potentially destructive ways. Expressing these emotions deliberately will ultimately result in relief and movement through the phases toward a better life.

You've got to make time every day, even if it's only a little bit of time, to express your losses. It may seem impossible, but structuring time for grieving needs to be part of your basic daily ADLs. Typically the kinds of healing activities you're going to do are personal enrichment activities, and I'll go into this in more detail in later phases. But in the crisis phase, it's important for you to treat grieving as a life-supportive ADL. At this point, expressing grief, loss, and fear is as necessary for you as eating or dressing. When people don't make time for grief, fear, and anger, these emotions make their own time. They may express themselves in the kind of uncontrolled talk or crying I mentioned earlier. They may also fuel aggression and anxiety attacks.

What do you actually do to express your feeling of fear, grief, and loss? First, you need to find and identify these feelings. You've probably been suppressing them as much as possible in order to get along. To find them, you need to quiet your mind of everyday things and let the feelings come forth. Some people get into this state of openness to what they're feeling by listening to music, meditating, or praying. These activities tune down the outside world and allow you to sense the ideas and feelings that daily activities drown out. Some people write in a journal and discover as they write that they're preoccupied with certain fears or angers or griefs or losses. Some people read other people's works and recognize their own feelings of fear or anger or grief in the author's expressions.

You should understand that allowing yourself this daily expression, though it's sometimes painful, can also be immediately relieving. Acknowledging or recognizing that this is how you feel permits your feelings to become real. They are real, but you haven't allowed yourself to see that before. You then express the emotions that the feelings produce. You may cry or sob or moan over your grief and your losses. You may rage—literally talk angrily, scream, or stomp around—about your angers. You may clutch a pillow, quilt, or large stuffed animal to your body in response to your fears. Any action or expression that doesn't hurt you or anyone else is fine. Do it. Even if these activities don't seem to relieve you, these purposeful actions will nonetheless help reduce the number of uncontrolled, spontaneous expressions of grief, fear, or anger that you may have found inappropriate or embarrassing.

Some people worry that if they begin expressing their grief or anger they'll never stop. Don't worry. You're only going to spend a limited amount of time each day actively working with them, perhaps twenty minutes once or twice a day. At first, if you haven't been expressing your emotions at all, you may want and need to spend a little more time doing so. Your counselor can help you work out how much time to spend. If you're spending more than half an hour crying or raging, contact your counselor. Clinical support can be very helpful at this time, so you should seek it out if you've got any questions or concerns about these necessary emotional exercises.

After you've begun performing daily "expressive" ADLs, you by yourself or you and your counselor should start to review what you've done in this area. You should start to build genuine insight into what is happening to you, what you feel, and what you're able to do about it. Greater insight will help you achieve better management of your crisis situation. When you give yourself this daily time, it will ultimately provide you with additional energy for other tasks since you'll no longer be using up precious energy trying to keep these feelings at bay.

When You Must Get Professional Help

If you're not already seeing a mental-health clinician and find yourself in deep water emotionally, you must talk with one. Your health-care team leader may be the person you turn to, or the team leader can refer you to an appropriate person. Deep trouble may take the form of crying uncontrollably several times a day, turning to anodynes like drugs or alcohol, or contemplating suicide.

Learning about the Phases

Now is the time to look at the journey ahead. Think about Betty's story and read through the phase chapters in this book. They'll help affirm your illness and trauma experience as well as your experience of loss and grief. You'll see how the phases function as a map so that you can locate where you are in the current moment. As you proceed through the phases, your sense of calm will increase because you'll be able to see in which direction you're going. You'll see that you and your loved ones are moving toward a better future that you can actually hope to attain.

Building Insight about Your Private Self.

As you carry out your expressive ADLs and discuss them with your counselor, you'll find that you're beginning to build understanding. Part of that understanding is the recognition that your private self—that young self—

serves a very important function during the crisis phase. In fact, that young self has a positive value. Even though your private self may have embarrassed you in public places or made you feel like you don't recognize yourself anymore, it has actually helped you by communicating to you and possibly to others what you couldn't otherwise imagine, let alone articulate. You may think you're managing, but your private self insists on demonstrating that you're actually afraid, in pain, confused, angry, and in need of help and comfort.

The private self was usually formed when you were young. As a result, it doesn't have the polish, the discrimination, and the differentiation that your grown-up public self has. Your private self may be more emotional than you're comfortable with. Nonetheless, you need to come to see that this aspect of yourself is basic, straightforward, and universal. We all have a private self. Whether we're chronically ill or not, we have all had to come to terms with a private self that we're sometimes ashamed of.

You may have heard this private self being called your "defenses" or your "child ego state." Whatever you call it, that part of yourself is now feeling overwhelmed, which is why it's intruding into your public life. But in response you don't want to ignore it, and you certainly don't want to try to suppress it, even if you could. Instead, you need to listen to it, be kind to it, become its ally. First of all, your private self is teaching you very basically and authentically how you feel, how you're suffering, how you feel under attack.

As you allow this aspect of yourself to emerge in your daily expressive ADLs, you gain insight into truths about your situation. Not only does this help you manage your crisis, but with the aid of your counselor you can also start "growing up" this authentic child self. As you move through the phases and learn to live meaningfully with chronic illness, you will eventually integrate this old private self into the new, mature self you create.

Learning How to Observe

To carry out your expressive ADLs and to learn the story of your unique illness experience, you need to become a good observer. It's a *crucial* skill. If you can't see yourself—if you can't name the thoughts, feelings, and behaviors of your private and public selves—you can't change and evolve as a person. By becoming an observer, you can stand apart from your suffering, frantic, personal self who's taken over most of your life in this crisis phase, and look at your daily life objectively. At the same time, you'll come to regard yourself and your life with compassion. Your counselor can help you learn observation skills. I'll be going into more depth on observation in later phases, but here in the crisis phase you want to begin learning how to accurately note and report information about your activities and your symptoms. Your counselor can help you learn by asking questions about the material you've collected. Sometimes you learn about things you've left out because you hadn't realized they were important. You may not have thought, for example, that making the bed was important. You may not have mentioned that you opened all the mail in the afternoon and sorted out the junk from the bills. The counselor's questions can also help you learn to distinguish degrees of difficulty you're having with symptoms. All of this observation is objective. The time that you got up in the morning is a fact. Whether you're able to dress yourself every day is a fact. Whether you drove to work is a fact. That you feel fatigue is a fact. That the fatigue you feel in the morning is worse than the evening is a fact.

As you and your counselor discuss the activities of your weekly life, you also will begin to learn to differentiate thoughts, feelings, and behaviors. What you think or feel about getting up or driving to work or being bone-tired can be teased apart from the facts of these things, but your understanding of your thoughts and feelings can become objective fact also. This can make them less painful to think and talk about. You learn how to stand outside yourself, looking in.

Some people learn to develop observational skills by themselves through meditation. They note all the thoughts that flow thought their minds as they attempt to empty their minds and thereby locate some of their persistent concerns and preoccupations. In general, however, it's best to work in concert with a professional to develop observational skills when you are in crisis.

Telling Your Own Story

It's crucially important for you to tell your own story and what's happening to you. You should not try to understand these things according to other people's interpretations and assessments. Hence you need to begin writing or otherwise creating your own life story immediately.

At first it may be hard for you to write things down. You may never have written anything in the past and you may not think you can. If that's the case, draw pictures with maybe a word or phrase to say what's important about the picture. Maybe you can begin your story by collecting objects that represent or recall different moments that are important in your life. Whatever form you use at first to begin telling your story, it usually helps you focus if you mentally divide your life into seven-year periods. Eventually you'll want to try to write down these memorable events, people, or places because a written record is easier to work with. As you go through the phases and develop new insights, you're going to revise your story.

Remember, it doesn't matter whether other people would think the things that you note down are important. It only matters that you think so. You write down both good and bad things, then move on to the next seven-year period. Eventually you arrive at your illness and your story of that illness. Again, it's not what other people think or what the media thinks, it's what *you* think that's important. Over time, you're actually going to rewrite this story of illness, but this records your first impressions and how you feel about it now.

Exercise 8, "Starting Your Story," will help you begin the brainstorming process. It gives you a chance to "see" different blocks of time in your life and to note down events and feelings that were important to you. Under

"Family," for instance, you may note that you had a particularly warm relationship with a sister or brother. Or perhaps you fought constantly with one of them or were very jealous of one. Maybe your mother or father was ill when you were young. Perhaps your parents divorced at that time. Maybe your parents fought all the time, or a stepfather behaved violently and scared you. In your teenage years, you may have had sexual experiences that changed your life. Maybe you played on a team where the coach was a particularly important mentor whose training has stayed with you ever since. Perhaps you had painful experiences with drugs or alcohol. When you were growing up, you may have hoped that you would become an astronaut or a singer. Maybe you dreamed about traveling all over the world. You may have loved the area in which you grew up or hated it. Maybe you never lived long enough in one place to ever feel at home. As a young man or woman, you may have made some friends who are still as close to you as anyone in your life. Parents, grandparents, siblings, or friends may have died during any of these periods.

In brainstorming and creating your story, use anything that helps you—photos, pictures from magazines, sketches you draw yourself. It's not important to use the actual paper form for Exercise 8. Simply let it help you organize your thoughts for now. Remember, you are going to be rethinking your story throughout your phase journey. This is not the last word on your narrative. There is no right or wrong, but only what you think now.

Working with Others

Illness Involves Others

You haven't gotten sick in isolation, and how your family, friends, and co-workers act makes a great difference in your experience of illness. Some of these people may not believe that you are sick at all, or not sick with a legitimate illness. If they do think you're sick, they may react with fear, anger, or sometimes even revulsion. Family members in particular may be ashamed or embarrassed about your condition, and they may resent the fact that you're sick. It means they have to do many of the things you used to do, and they keep having to make excuses about you to others. Even if they are understanding, their behavior may make life difficult for you. They may try to control you and what you do about your condition rather than letting you determine how you will handle your illness.

Exercise 9, "You and Your Family," will help you clarify how your family is reacting to your chronic illness. In Exercise 9, it's important for you to be specific about how you know that family members have the attitudes they do. For example, your father may be very understanding about your condition, which he shows by asking you intelligent questions. He may show that he's not controlling by, on the one hand, exhibiting an interest and concern (demonstrated by questions to you), but, at the same time, not taking control

Exercise 8
Starting Your Story

	Family	Friends	School/Work	Sex/Partners	Health	Hopes/Plans	Troubles/Fears
Birth to 7 years							
7 to 14 years							
14 to 21 years							
21 to 28 years							
28 to 35 years*							

* Add age ranges as necessary

Exercise 9
You and Your Family

Belief and Understanding

1. Do family members believe what you say about yourself and your illness?

   Which members believe you?

   How do you know? Describe instances that show their attitude.

   Which members don't believe you?

   How do you know? Describe instances that show their attitude.

2. Do family members understand your illness?

   Which members understand?

   How do you know they do?

   Which members don't understand?

   How do you know they don't?

Shame, Embarrassment, Resentment

1. Are family members embarrassed by your illness or ashamed?

   Which members are embarrassed?

   How do you know they are?

2. Are family members resentful of your illness?

   Which members are resentful?

   How do you know they are?

Control Issues

1. Do family members try to control your illness or your treatment?

> If family members try to control your behavior, give instances of how they do.

> If family members let you run your illness, give instances of how they demonstrate this.

Family Losses and Suffering

1. Do family members express loss or suffering because of your illness?

> Which family members show loss or suffering?

> How do they show they feel this way?

---

by saying what course of action you should take or criticizing either your treatment plan or how you're following it. As another example, your spouse is invited to the company picnic. You aren't capable of going and your spouse doesn't want to go without you. If he or she calls up to say that you both will not be coming because you have a condition that makes it impossible, your spouse is demonstrating a lack of embarrassment or shame. If, however, he or she says that you can't come because of prior commitments or because you'll be out of town, then he or she is feeling some embarrassment about your condition.

Family and Friends Suffer, Too

Try to remember that your family, your friends, and even your co-workers suffer because of your illness. Your illness hurts them in a variety of ways by depriving them of the person you used to be before you got sick. Because you may be suffering many traumas yourself, it's sometimes hard to pay much attention to other people's losses. The issue here is not for you to feel guilty, but for you to be aware of the sufferings of others and to try to understand them. Otherwise it will be very difficult for you to work together with these important people to make your life better.

Couples Issues

If you have a spouse or a partner, several issues are important right away. Sexual activity often becomes difficult or impossible for patients with a chronic illness because you just don't feel like it at all. Distribution of jobs and responsibilities often changes abruptly because you can't do many (maybe most) of the things you used to. And sometimes finances become a serious concern if you are missing a lot of work or can't work at all.

In the crisis phase, most couples manage to deal with the special circumstances of a partner's illness if it doesn't last too long. The real work usually comes in phase two. But if the onset of your chronic illness has taken place over a long period of time, your partner can be getting pretty angry and hurt about living with this new situation long-term.

The relationship between a couple is so important and so emotionally charged that it often helps to have someone act as a helper and a guide toward understanding the new situation. Your health-care team leader may be able to help you navigate these uncharted waters or can recommend a counselor or couples therapist if necessary. If you have a very strong and open relationship, you may be able to do some work on your own.

Exercise 10, "You and Your Partner," gives you a way to examine some of the major issues that most couples face. You and your partner should each fill out a copy, then compare your assessments and discuss your understandings with each other. The issues examined in Exercise 9 also apply to couples.

Family Issues

You may have children who are having difficulty adjusting to the new you. Or, if you are single, you may have been forced by your illness to move back with your parents. You may never have left home. In addition, you probably have relatives—aunts, uncles, cousins—who are reacting to you in a variety of ways. They may need trauma education, and your team leader can probably recommend helpful books or offer to speak with them.

The age of children makes a lot of difference in how you explain to them why things are different, but you need to help them try to understand what is happening in their world. If you are an adult living again with parents, it can be very hard to explain what's happening. Issues of control can also become particularly difficult if you've returned to your parents' home. However, as with couples issues, phase one is often a time when other people in your life try to accommodate to the new situation. It is only when the situation goes on—when it becomes what they perceive as chronic—that the most serious difficulties arise. Hence you'll probably do most of your family and living companion work in phase two.

Friendships

Many adults with chronic illness choose to live with a friend, in which case many of the issues relating to family and couples apply. No matter where you're living and whom you live with, if anyone, you'll probably need to work out issues of control, roles and responsibilities, and so forth.

Exercise 10
You and Your Partner

Roles and Responsibilities

1. What were your roles and responsibilities before you became ill?

2. What are your roles and responsibilities since you became ill?

3. Are you and your partner in agreement about your changed roles and responsibilities?

> Have you spoken together about the changes or have the changes simply occurred without comment?

> What do you think should be done differently?

Finances

1. Has your illness changed your financial picture as a couple?

> What are the changes?

2. Do you and your partner discuss financial issues?

> About what do you agree?

> About what do you disagree?

Sex

1. How has your sex life been affected by your illness?

2. Can you and your partner speak candidly about the changing sexual picture?

3. Have you found satisfactory ways to express sexuality in this new situation?

Emotions

1. Is your partner angry because of your condition?

    If so, how is this expressed?

2. Is your partner expressing loss because of your condition?

    If so, how is this apparent to you?

3. Is your partner expressing suffering because of your condition?

    If so, how is this apparent to you?

Companionability

1. How did you used to spend time together before you became ill?

2. How do you spend time together since you became ill?

3. Do you enjoy talking to each other?

4. How has your relationship with each other changed since you became ill?

It's sometimes hard to realize that you're still worth being someone's friend when you're feeling that nothing of the old you remains. It doesn't help that some of your friends stay far away from you once they realize that you're sick. It's a sad fact that many people can't deal with illness or are frightened by it. In time you may be able to reincorporate some of these people into your social life, but most people with chronic illness find that they lose some old friends forever.

Remember that you can be ill and still be a friend. It's just that how you do it may change. Friends are people who share their lives with you, who listen and care about your life, and who enjoy your company. You may not be able to do some of the active physical things you used to or even go out to lunch. But you can still talk and listen and care. Naturally, when you're caught up in the crisis of your illness onset, it's hard to think of much except yourself. But to maintain a friendship you've got to give equal time to your friends' concerns. And you have to be careful not to overload any one friend with too much about your illness. When you find a friend who's willing (even anxious) to listen to all your woes, you usually want to talk to them constantly. But they'll burn out if you do that. You can also learn how to arrange when you visit with friends (whether by email, phone, or in person) so that you don't exhaust yourself. Exercise 11, "You and Your Friends," asks you questions about how you act with friends, which will give you some insight into what you're actually doing. Remember, if you're living with a friend, you want to review Exercises 9 and 10 to see if any of those questions apply.

Work Issues

Your illness may have forced you to leave work altogether, but many chronically ill people, especially in the crisis phase, still try to go to work full- or part-time. If you're still working, you've probably discovered that some of your co-workers or your supervisor are becoming annoyed because of the sick time you've taken, the fact that you can't meet deadlines or keep up your old pace of work, or because you come in late and leave early a lot.

For obvious reasons, many people do not want to inform the workplace about their illness. But you may have to say something or it may become known anyway. In any case, there are a number of things you can do to help make your work situation better. The Americans with Disabilities Act requires employers to meet certain needs of people whose condition interferes with their ability to complete their job in the traditional fashion. You can investigate part-time work with your present employer or a flexible schedule that would allow you to do some work at home. You may be able to move onto temporary disability so as not to exhaust your sick leave. As with many things about chronic illness, your options vary depending on where you work and what the company policies are.

Again, you'll probably find yourself managing somehow during the crisis phase. It's usually in phase two that most chronic illness patients begin to

Exercise 11
You and Your Friends

1. Do you see or have contact with your old friends?

   Whom do you still see?

   Whom don't you see any longer?

   Why?

2. How do you visit with friends (by phone, letter, e-mail, in person)?

3. What do you talk about when you see friends?

   Do you talk about your illness or how you're feeling?
   What percentage of the conversation?

   Do you talk about what your friends are doing?
   What percentage of the conversation?

   Are you interested in the things that your friends have to say?
   If yes, why?

   If no, why?

   Are your friends interested in your current issues and activities?
   How do they show they interest?

4. Do you ask your friends for help?
   What kinds of help do you request?

   Which friends do you ask help from?

Exercise 12
Work Issues

1. Are you working at the same job that you were working at before becoming ill?

2. Are you working the same number of hours a week?

3. Has your illness become an issue with your employer?

    Because of sick leave taken?

    Because of work not completed?

    Because of health-care costs?

    Because of fear of your illness?

    Other reasons?

4. Do your co-workers or colleagues have issues with your illness?

    Are they resentful?
        Why?

    Are they fearful?
        Why?

    Are they supportive?
        How do they show it?

5. Is your job now difficult for you?

    Because of the commute to work?

    Because of physical conditions at the workplace?

    Because of fatigue?

    Because of cognitive difficulties?

    Other reasons (specify)?

reorganize their work arrangements intentionally. If, however, you need help with your employment situation immediately, call upon your health-care team leader. This person can provide the workplace with advice and conduct the interventions that you require, or will help locate a professional who can assist you. Workplace interventions include assessing your work environment to see whether it can be rearranged to reduce stress, speaking with your employer about the nature of your illness and your capacity to continue working, and conducting information training with your co-workers to reduce their fears and stigmatization of you. If you can't continue to work, this advisor can help guide you through the process of applying for disability. If you're still working, fill out Exercise 12, "Work Issues." It will give you a way to assess where you are now with regard to work.

Advocacy Role of Your Health-Care Team Leader

It's the job of at least one member of your health-care team, usually your team leader, not only to provide the care you need, but also to speak for your needs and interests in the outside world. This is why you should put together a team in whom you have the greatest confidence. You should believe in their competence and trust them, but it is equally important that you *like* them, particularly the team leader. Your team leader must be willing to help you find the resources you need and be readily sympathetic to your concerns. Exercise 13, "You and Your Health-Care Team," asks questions that will help you decide if you've put together a good health-care team.

Coping and Comfort

Relationships

Strong, supportive relationships are key to moving forward through the illness phases. You need to have people who understand your situation and who care about you. You need people who can help you solve practical problems, achieve the insights you need to approach a better life, and give you a sympathetic place to grieve for your losses and suffering. If you're fortunate, you have a supportive family and many friends. But it's sufficient if you have just a couple of good friends to provide the necessary support. Professionals also have special skills and resources to offer, and extensive experience with others who have been through your experience. Few individuals with chronic illness can travel the long journey of their illness without the aid of a truly caring health-care team leader. Take a few minutes now to write down the names of those people among your family, friends, or health-care professionals who can be part of the supportive group.

Comfort Areas

While in the crisis of phase one, it's extremely important for you to make your bunker retreat as comfortable as possible. You probably won't be able to

Exercise 13
You and Your Health-Care Team

1. Do you have a primary-care physician?

   What are this person's qualifications?

   Does this person listen to you carefully?

   Does this person treat you with respect?

   Does this person discuss any issues about your condition with you or refer you to professionals who can help?

2. Do you have a good relationship with your primary care physician's office staff?

3. Have you identified a health-care team leader?

   Is this person capable of spending the time with you that you need?

   What are this person's qualifications?

   Does this person listen to you carefully?

   Does this person treat you with respect?

   Does this person help you keep track of and understand all your tests, medications, treatments?

   Does this person make sure that protocols ordered by various clinicians don't interfere with or contradict each other?

4. Have you been given a referral to a counselor?

   What are this person's qualifications?

   Is this person someone you trust and like?

   Does this person listen to you carefully and treat you with respect?

do this alone, either because you're not physically capable of it or because you don't live alone and you need to have the agreement and participation of the other people living with you. A counselor is particularly useful here because these professionals can teach you how to go about getting the help you need from others. They also make it possible for you to practice new roles before you've got to use them in your regular life.

First, you'll want to make the overall environment comfortable. This includes paying attention to all five senses—sight, sound, smell, touch, and taste. You'll also want to arrange certain personal comforts. You'll want to select people you can rely on—safe people—to be your companions during this intense period. And you'll want to arrange for certain emotional comforts, which include some spiritual or philosophical supports.

Environmental Comforts

The place you go to be safe, your bunker, must be comfortable and easy to keep clean and attractive. If you live by yourself, this may include your entire apartment, but if you have a partner or a family, you may be limited to your bedroom or a space that is yours alone. Perhaps there isn't any space that will be wholly your own. In that case, you have to try to create spaces in rooms you share with others and establish certain ground rules, especially with regard to noise. Where negotiations of this sort are difficult, you can call upon your counselor for help.

Light is extremely important. I recommend no overhead, harsh lighting, but indirect lighting that can be raised or lowered easily. Noise tends to tire chronically ill people. Your special space should be as far as possible from family noise. You need to negotiate limits with regard to how loud talking, music, TV, or videos will be. You should have a bed or share a bed that has a surface beside it on which you can put food and liquid. In addition to a bed, you need a reclining place (probably a sofa or a reclining chair), and it, too, should have an easily accessible surface next to it on which you can put food and liquids. If possible, you should have a TV and VCR in the room where you can recline. You should also have a work station—a desk and chair, perhaps with a computer—that is yours alone. If you have one particular room, it should have whatever curtains, pictures, and rugs that are pleasing to you, but you should have as few decorative objects or other clutter as possible. You want this space to be a cinch to keep neat and clean. Consider this space as your birdcage in the sense that you want to be able to change the paper at the bottom really easily. If you share all spaces in your dwelling with others, try to make those items you use particularly easy to keep clean and neat.

Outside your special space or spaces, you also need to consider whether you need other items. Do you need a chair in the shower so that you can sit while washing? Do you need a handrail in the bathtub or beside the toilet? Do you need a stool in the kitchen to sit on while preparing food or washing dishes? Do you need a food cart so you don't have to carry items from the stove to the table? Do you need handrails elsewhere in the house? In phase two, after your condition has stabilized, you may ask your health-care team leader to bring in a physical therapist or an occupational therapist to make a professional assessment of your physical living arrangements.

Personal Comforts

Make sure that you have comfortable, loose, cozy clothing to wear when you're not in public. The clothing should be whatever makes you feel physically pampered. You shouldn't have to wear a bra, a belt, stockings, a tie, or anything constricting. If the seams of clothing or the labels at the back of the neck bother you, go ahead and wear the clothes inside out. In other words, you should have available clothing that actually makes you feel good and cared for. In addition, try to acquire one set of comfortable but presentable clothes to wear in public. These should require as little effort to get into as possible and should be easy to keep. For instance, these clothes should be machine washable and not require any ironing.

You should also identify simple snack foods and beverages that you particularly like. Try to avoid things that can make your condition worse—alcohol being a major one. The point is to have a small quantity of foods that you really like so that you can increase your sense of caring for yourself by snacking on these treats while you read or watch TV.

Keep a tape player beside your bed with relaxing tapes (music, mood or atmospheric tapes) or a radio tuned to a quiet talk show, in case you wake at night. You also want to have water by your bedside and some crackers or fruit in case you're hungry when you wake.

You can make a schedule of TV shows that you enjoy and get a video-store card so that you can rent movies to watch. If possible, you should subscribe to cable TV. If you like to read, have a variety of books available—some serious, some totally escapist. There should be no censorship here. If you like bodice-ripper romances or techno-thrillers, get some. If you like children's adventure books, get them. If you like mysteries, collect a stack. Your effort here is to make your bunker a place you like, a place in which you can truly relax and, insofar as possible, forget your problems altogether.

People Comforts

It's hard to keep up friendships when you're experiencing the crisis of chronic illness onset. You've got so much else on your mind that when you're with friends, you can talk pretty single-mindedly about your own problems or else be secretly distracted by them. Often what your friends have to say makes you angry or envious because you're not participating in those things anymore. Sometimes their interests can just seem empty to you in your condition. Some people don't want to burden their friends with their troubles. But it is crucially important for you to talk about what's happening to you. It's also important for you to listen to your friends and respond to their concerns and interests.

Human warmth is important. You need to make an effort to stay in touch with people who believe you, believe in your illness, and want to support you and comfort you. You can't just dump your woes on them, though. Consciously make yourself exercise proper friendship etiquette by asking them about themselves and their lives and really listening to their replies. In addition to being the friendly thing to do, their stories can also distract you. You may even be giving your friend something valuable that they really need—a willing ear. For chronic illness patients, being a good and sympathetic listener can often make up profoundly for not being able to get out for more physical activities with friends.

If your onset crisis keeps you at home all the time, try to have daily contact with another person in one way or another. This could include medical people, business or service people, and acquaintances. At least every other day, you should be in contact with a good friend or relative, either by e-mail or phone. At least once a week you should actually see someone. It's best to try to see a variety of people so that you don't become dependent on any one person. If you don't spread out your contact, your one person may easily burn out under the intensity of your need. Your counselor can help you figure out who would be good for you to see and how to make it happen.

Spiritual and Philosophical Comforts

Many people in the crisis phase of chronic illness feel spiritually abandoned. They feel it's their fault that they're sick and that God is punishing them, has abandoned them, or doesn't exist at all. I absolutely refuse to believe that you are being punished, but these feelings are not uncommon among new chronic illness patients. It seems to be an almost automatic, organic response to the shame that your illness and the society's reaction to your illness produces. In the first wretchedness of chronic illness, it's hard not to feel that life is meaningless. At first, you'll probably have to go on sheer faith—mine, if no one else's—but you aren't going to stay in this grim place forever.

With your counselor, you'll need to begin trying to express your feelings of fear, anger, suffering, and loss. You're permitted to say that you're suffering, to express that suffering, and to feel sorrow about your losses. You can *allow* your suffering to exist even though you didn't ask for it and didn't want it. Remember, this genuine expression of feeling is necessary to your healing. The task of allowing its existence is necessary in order to move forward.

You can also begin to share with some trusted others how you feel about the fact that your illness is hard to get a handle on. You can talk about what it feels like to be sick with something that goes on and on.

Your counselor can also teach you some techniques for making calmness in the midst of all the crisis and chaos you're experiencing. You can learn meditation and relaxation techniques. You can listen to soothing tapes. If you're a reader, there are books that may help to anchor you. And, most important, you can devote some time to your own story, to creating the record of who you were, what happened, and where you're going as each day goes by.

When you're in crisis, it doesn't seem like any of this will help. Trust me—*it will help*. For now you need to accept the faith and experience of others that what you're experiencing is normal for people with chronic conditions and that you will feel differently as time goes on. Your situation can change for the better.

Forward from Crisis

In phase one, your goal is containment of the crisis. You do this by putting together a health-care team you can rely on and by making sure you're safe physically. With one member of your health-care team you form a strong, trusting, caring bond, and together you begin shoring up support for yourself psychologically. With this helper, you affirm the reality of your illness, your hurts or traumas, and your losses, and you begin to express grief for them. You learn about the nature of chronic illnesses and the phases that you will pass through on the way to achieving a better, meaningful life. You also learn how to observe your activities and feelings objectively so that you can stop sabotaging yourself and begin organizing your energies most effectively. Finally, you begin the process of establishing new relationships with the other people in your life. With the help of your counselor, you also deal with pressing workplace issues if necessary.

You're now moving into phase two, the stabilization phase, which I'll discuss in the next chapter. You've weathered the crisis and have regained a bit of control over your existence by cutting back to the simplest life you can. Now, slowly and gradually, you're going to begin restructuring your overall life. You're going to start to discover the actual physical boundaries of your new life so that you can keep yourself as healthy as possible and avoid precipitating relapses. You're going to develop your observational and interpretative skills even more fully so that you can truly understand your situation and begin establishing a new set of norms and values for living. And you're going to continue working with others so that your social world becomes more supportive.

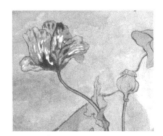

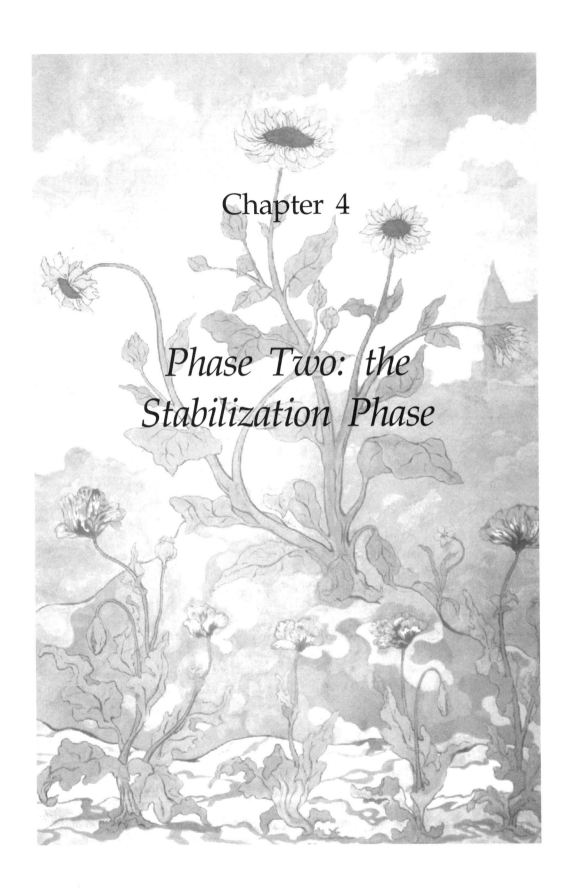

Chapter 4

Phase Two: the Stabilization Phase

Stabilization

How can you tell when you've moved from the crisis phase into the stabilization phase? Certain changes in how you feel make this pretty clear.

You feel greater control. Time has passed since you experienced the crisis of your illness starting. Maybe you now have a diagnosis for your condition. But even if you don't, you probably have discovered a sort of pattern in how you experience your illness. You don't like it, but you've gotten used to it. You've learned some ways to cope, so life doesn't seem as desperate as it did when you first got sick.

You've begun seeking. You're looking for all sorts of things. Mostly you're looking for people who understand and support you. If your illness has been diagnosed, you've probably gotten in touch with the local support group for your illness or at least thought about it. You may have gone online to look for information about the condition and to find chat rooms of people like yourself. If you hear about people with your illness, maybe you get in touch with them.

You may also be looking for more satisfactory health care. You may not feel that your regular practitioner is up to handling your illness. Perhaps you feel that the specialists you've seen haven't helped you very much either. But you believe that effective treatment is out there somewhere, if only you could find it.

You don't blame yourself quite so much anymore. When you first recognized that something was wrong with you, you may have felt that somehow you'd brought it on yourself. Something about you being you was making you suffer all these strange symptoms. Now you probably think this way a little less. You believe that you have an illness the way people with pneumonia have an illness. It's just that no one seems to know very much about your illness, or else the people you've seen don't seem to be doing much to cure it.

You're having fewer repetitive, disturbing thoughts. When you first got sick, some ideas or scenes probably kept replaying themselves over and over in your mind. For some people who feel very bad, these thoughts are about death or suicide. But these repetitive thoughts gradually diminish as you enter phase two.

You don't deny that you're sick so much of the time. One way that some people deal with the crisis of getting sick is to pretend to themselves that they aren't sick. They're really fine, it's just that today was a very bad day, and maybe yesterday was bad as well. Everybody has some bad days, you think. Usually events during the crisis stage have forced you to acknowledge that something's wrong, and you go to see a doctor. But even if you receive a diagnosis, you may keep telling yourself that you're not really sick.

You're just tired or very stressed. In phase two, however, most of the time you acknowledge that you're ill.

You're sick and tired of this problem going on and on. During the crisis phase, you were probably preoccupied with how you felt. You wanted to get the problem diagnosed and treated just as you would want a case of pneumonia diagnosed and treated. But even after the health-care people diagnosed you (if they have) and gave you various treatments to help with your symptoms, you are still sick. Maybe the symptoms have been relieved or are better some of the time, but the problem has not gone away. Your doctor has probably told you that you've got a chronic illness. But it's just now sinking in what "chronic" means. It means something that goes on indefinitely. And you're not buying into that. You want a cure.

Strategy: Living the Enforced Monastic Life

Goal. The goal in phase two is to stabilize and begin restructuring your life. The strategy for attaining this goal is what I call "living the enforced monastic life." I don't mean by this that you've got to take a vow of poverty, chastity, or obedience, even though sometimes your illness and the fallout from it makes you feel like you have. I mean that in this phase you're going to lead a very conscious, structured life, where you pay close attention to what you do and how you do it. This is going to help you stabilize. You also need to learn to find satisfaction in performing small, often humble tasks.

Once again you're going to accomplish this strategy through tactics and skills aimed at the three different but interconnected parts of your life: your physical self, your psychological self, and yourself as you relate to others.

Learning your new physical boundaries. You're going to start discovering the new boundaries of what you can do in life. These may have changed radically since you got sick. You need to know how to locate these new physical boundaries and how to select daily and weekly activities so you have the most complete, fulfilling life possible.

Regrouping psychologically. Now that you've survived the crisis of phase one, you're able to reflect in a more thoughtful way about yourself and what's happened. You first need to learn how to examine your life so that your thinking is helpful and productive. Then, as you begin to understand yourself and your new situation, you start constructing a set of norms and values for living the new life that you're in now.

Working with the reactions of others. Just as your attitudes and feelings have changed since your illness first began, so have those of the people around you. Like you, they're beginning to experience your illness as a chronic thing, not an emergency that's going to go away when you get better.

Even in phase one some people in your life began to line up on a continuum, but in phase two practically everyone you know does. At one end are people who believe in your illness and who will try their best to help and support you. At the other end are those who don't buy your illness at all and who suspect that you're lazy or crazy and not worth the trouble. Most people—whether family, friends, co-workers, acquaintances, even health-care practitioners—fall somewhere in between these two extremes.

Tactics and Skills

Learning Your New Physical Boundaries

Checkups with your medical team. Most people entering phase two have reached a plateau of symptoms. This means that even though you still have symptoms, often serious and debilitating ones, they're fairly predictable and you're familiar with them. Sometimes your medications or other medical protocols help relieve them, but sometimes you just know their pattern so you're not as scared. You have found ways to cope or just hang in with your symptoms. A plateau may last for a long time. You may even improve. But with chronic illness, you may also suffer a relapse. So it's very important for you to check in regularly with your medical team. When you achieve a plateau, particularly the first time, you should consult with your medical team. They may want to adjust your medications or recommend other therapies.

Review medications. You may have been given medications when you first got sick that were intended to reduce the severity of your symptoms. When you reach a plateau, that goal has been accomplished. The health-care team may now want to reduce you to a maintenance dose or perhaps eliminate some medications altogether. They may want to switch you to an entirely different set of medications.

Introduce other therapies. Now that you're out of crisis, your physical condition may have improved enough for you to tolerate a different set of medical protocols. You may now be able to benefit from physical or occupational therapy, where before you probably couldn't physically or psychologically take on anything else.

Readjusting your physical activities. An essential activity in phase two is for you to reexamine all the activities you used to do or wanted to do. You'll then categorize these activities so that when you begin selecting the activities that will be part of your new life, you can make sure to include activities from each major category. But first, you need to learn about the personal energy process.

Personal energy process (PEP). When performing an action, everyone goes through a cycle. At the start of the action, you feel a little or a lot of resistance. It can be like trying to roll a stone or a boulder. But once you've begun doing whatever the action is (paying a bill, typing a memo, changing a faucet washer), it usually moves along pretty smoothly. It's like when your car shifts into high gear and just rolls down the highway. At completion of the action, if you still have energy left, you feel a physical sense of satisfaction in addition to an emotional one. We all need to complete this process many times a day for us to have a healthy sense of emotional and physical well-being.

Impaired PEP cycle. When you've got a chronic illness and haven't developed new activity boundaries, you can easily exhaust yourself and fail to complete PEP cycles properly. You may be able to finish an action, but you're so physically drained that you get no sense of fulfillment, only a sense of bone-weariness. Or maybe you can't complete the activity you started at all, and you feel a debilitating sense of failure.

This happens to healthy people as well as to the chronically ill, but it's more likely to happen to people with a chronic illness. When you're chronically ill, you may often want to pass as being healthy and capable. Maybe you don't want to have to explain about your illness, or maybe you think others have already cut you as much slack as they're willing to. Perhaps you just want to believe that you're healthy, or at least capable of doing a particular simple action. Whatever the reason, you end up pushing yourself too far and either fail or suffer exhaustion. Then you feel worse than you did before attempting the activity. If you accumulate many such failures, you're going to begin to feel really bad about yourself.

Basic constitution. In the last chapter I talked about people having a basic physical constitution. As you begin to restructure your activities, you need to give serious thought to what your basic constitution was before you got sick. If in the past you couldn't do many different things in a day or do them swiftly, then your restructured activities should take into consideration that you were not an enormously active person to begin with.

Four categories of activity. In the last chapter I also mentioned the four broad categories of life activities. In phase one, you needed to concentrate on the activities of daily living (ADLs). But now that you've attained the greater stability of phase two, you need to consider all four categories: ADLs, personal-enrichment activities, socially interactive activities, and work activities.

Before selecting the activities you wish to include in your restructured daily life, you need to identify which category each of your present activities belongs to. Reexamine Exercise 3 from the last chapter. Try putting each activity into the grid of Exercise 14, "Your Activities by Activity Group." Remember that ADLs you do for yourself are ADLs, but when you perform those same tasks for someone else (husband, child, friend, housemate), they fall into the work category. Add activities that you want to do but perhaps

Exercise 14
Your Activities by Activity Group

Activities of Daily Living (ADLs)	Personal Enrichment Activities	Social Activities	Work Activities

were unable to do because your past schedule was too busy. You may find these among your "Desires" in Exercise 4. Then add the activities that your illness requires you to perform. Regular physical therapy visits, for example, and medical visits or protocols can absorb a considerable amount of time and energy, so they need to be included along with the other activities that will go into your restructured life. Exercise 14 should give you a picture, by category, of the things you did in your old life, the things you want to do, and the things you now have to do for your health.

Using your PEP cycle to determine how much you do. You now need to consider how much energy you have each day because you're going to try putting more activities back into your life. What boundaries do you need to draw around your restructured life? One way to begin thinking about this is to consider how much energy you have left after you perform the essential ADLs that were your main activities during phase one. Without thinking, you've begun doing additional things as you've felt better or more in control. If you're paying close attention to your life (as you need to be at this time), you know whether you've got a bit of energy left when you finish a task, at the end of the day, and at the end of the week. This means that the activities you're doing fit into your PEP cycle. If, however, you're getting exhausted and drained after tasks (or at the end of the day or week), then you've got to reexamine your activities again. You've probably taken on too many things in addition to your ADLs, or you've begun doing your ADLs in the old way, using more energy.

Differing capabilities. There's a big difference in physical capability among people with chronic illness. Maybe, for example, you're a person who can continue to go to a job where you still perform fairly effectively. But maybe you're not often capable of getting out of bed at all. Some chronic illnesses are far more debilitating than others, and some people have far more disabling symptoms of the same illness. Many people experience great fluctuations in their symptoms. Whatever your personal experience of your illness, the general principle holds. In phase one everyone needs to cut back to doing almost nothing except their ADLs and work activities, if they can. Some people may have difficulty completing even 50 percent of their ADLs. In phase two, everyone needs to consider each new activity they put back into their lives very carefully, whether they're bedridden or still going off to a job.

Adding activities. For every new activity you'd like to add to your life, think about the following: How much energy does it take? Do you feel exhausted when you've completed this activity? Does it fulfill a need for you which makes that expenditure of energy worthwhile? Are there other activities you'd prefer to spend the energy on? How do you feel at the end of the day? After you've tried including two or three more activities for a week, analyze how you feel at the end of the week. If you're feeling tired, depressed, or drained, you need to cut back again. You may have chosen several activities that all require a great deal of energy. Or you may have included too many activities even though individually they don't use up too much energy. Or, finally, you may have selected activities you don't want to perform but that other people want you to do.

Balanced activity modification. In the crisis phase you learned how to reduce your ADLs or rearrange them to use your energy more efficiently. You're now in the process of trying to modify all your activities to create a life that you can actually sustain. As you do this, it is essential to include activities from all four categories. If you're severely disabled by your illness, you may be unable to include any activities in the work category. But otherwise, it's important for your physical and emotional health to have some activities every day from all four categories.

If you're very restricted by your illness, you may have to continue to focus almost completely on your ADLs. If this is the case, it's even more important than it was in phase one for you to allow time for what I called your "expressive" ADLs. This is where you spend some time each day thinking quietly, meditating, reading, listening to music, praying, or telling your story in some fashion. It's crucial that you continue to engage in activities that will eventually help you begin to develop a sense of what this all means. The real work of meaning development comes in phase three, but you begin taking the first steps way back in phase one.

To help you build a realistic daily schedule, take a blank copy of Exercise 14 and experiment by making up a daily list of activities for your life as you're living it now. When you look at this new schedule, do you think you can complete these activities without exhausting yourself? Will you have some energy left over each day? This can be hard to judge by yourself. You are now drawing the new boundaries of your physical life, and it's important to arrive at a true estimation of your energy and capacity.

It is also important to remember that what you can do—what your physical boundaries are—will change over time. You need to pay attention and monitor your activities during each day. You have to consciously ask yourself whether you're keeping up with actions that will make a big overall difference in how you feel. Ask yourself periodically, "Do I need to sleep now? Do I need to eat? Do I need to urinate?" Check on how you're feeling. Ask yourself, "Am I getting tired? Am I getting confused? Are my symptoms getting worse?"

The daily activity structure you establish now is not for all time. It applies to you as you are at present. Carrying out this exercise once, however, will teach you how to do it in the future, when your capacity to act either grows or contracts.

Teamwork. I mentioned in chapter 2 how important teamwork was among your health-care team. But it's equally important for you to work as part of a team when you're trying to modify your life activities and set new physical boundaries. It's extremely hard to evaluate activities and make judgments about what's necessary in your life unless you've got someone to talk with about these issues. Perhaps you have a reliable, insightful friend whom you trust and who will work well with you. But it may be an even better idea to work with the social worker or occupational therapist on your health-care team. Social workers make it their business to understand the systems in people's lives, from relationships between housemates or family members to work issues. They have a lot of experience and may be able to make suggestions or raise issues that neither you nor your friends have thought of.

Regrouping Psychologically

Reviewing and revising your personal narrative. As you enter phase two, you feel that your life is becoming more stable and that you're a little more in control of things. Now is a good time to revisit the story you wrote about yourself during the crisis phase. Examine how you felt then about what happened, how your friends and family reacted, what your co-workers thought and did, how you felt your medical professionals treated you, and what you thought about the general attitude of society toward people with your kinds of problems. Do you have additional insights now? In what ways do you think that the attitudes you and your family originally had toward illness affected how you responded to the onset of your chronic illness? Have your experiences during your illness onset and now, as you enter phase two, changed any of your attitudes? Have they changed the attitudes of those around you? Revise your story, noting ways in which your new insights have been changing old attitudes.

Refining your skills of self-observation. In the crisis phase you began the process of self-observation as you started tracking your activities and symptoms and as you started to write your own story. In phase two you're going to develop these skills.

Process and content. A distinction exists between content and process in your life. "Content" includes all the different, individual things that you do over time. "Process" is the way in which you do these things. The content of your life may vary greatly, but your processes tend to be consistent. If you look carefully at how you do things, you will probably recognize themes that characterize how you act. How, for example, do you behave when you meet someone new? How do you relate to people? How do you handle conflict? How do you establish trust? You need to stand apart from yourself as you're thinking about your typical processes, and try to be as objective as possible. Try completing Exercise 15, "Content and Process," a couple of times using different events or encounters. This will help you to see the difference between content and process.

Exercise 15
Content and Process

Teasing Out Content

1. Describe an event or encounter specific to your illness.

2. In the form below, list **similar** situations in your past. Write in how you felt, what you thought, and what you did or how you behaved.

Situation	What I felt	What I thought	What I did
1.			
2.			
3.			

3. Now fill in the form for the current event or encounter.

Current Situation	What I felt	What I thought	What I did

Process

1. List the features common to all these events or encounters, past and present.

2. Generalize about how you feel, think, and behave in this kind of event or encounter.

Observing self. In phase one you were introduced to the idea of a neutral, observing self. That's you, but a you who can look at your suffering self's experience objectively but with compassion. You can also use this same observing self to see how you respond to new situations—what your process is—even though the content of the situation seems different from past experiences. And you can begin to assess whether your typical processes sometimes stand in the way of handling a situation effectively.

Identification and differentiation. Gradually your observing self needs to learn how to identify fears, interpersonal relations, losses, and suffering and how to differentiate experiences from each other. Begin by asking yourself how you feel. What is changing in your life? How diminished do you feel before the world at large? How do you feel privately, just by yourself, compared with the person you used to be?

Things in your life right now may often cause you heightened fear or a sense of loss because of events in your past. Maybe you remember how irritated your mother was when you had a serious illness as a child. Maybe you remember how strained the family finances were when your father was out of work for a year because of illness. Perhaps your parents divorced after your mother got breast cancer. Your memory of those past events makes you fear that you will suffer as badly or worse in the present situation. You need to separate past experiences from present ones and differentiate what things are truly related to one another and what things are not. Past emotions may not apply at all to the current situation. Differentiation also helps you break your experience into manageable parts that in turn make it easier to solve problems. Try completing Exercise 16, "Identification and Differentiation." This should help you learn to carry out the process of identification and differentiation.

Teamwork again! Even the most thoughtful people can have a hard time getting the knack of the observing self. When you're ready to begin the intense work of self-examination, it can make a great difference to have someone who can ask questions and draw attention to patterns in what you are saying. Once again you will probably benefit by having a counselor or a very insightful friend help you get started and maybe even continue with you in the process. Saying things out loud can also give them a reality that they don't have when you have the idea only in your head or only written on a piece of paper.

Overcoming psychological defenses. I talked briefly in phase one about the psychological defenses that everyone has as part of their private, often childlike self. These defenses serve a very important purpose in your life and have probably protected you from harm. But they can also stand in the way of your achieving a new and better way of living.

In addition, you've got a personality that affects how open you will be to new ways of thinking. You may, for example, be a generally cooperative person who likes to get along with others. You try to make sure that people will like and help you by telling them what you think they want to hear and by doing what you think they want you to do. But with a chronic illness, this can be very counterproductive for your health. People may be asking you to do things that you can't do without further damaging your health.

Maybe instead you've always been a vigorous, achieving person. You simply can't believe that you could have a condition that diminishes you. This kind of character can stand in the way of your making necessary adjustments in your life so that you will be able to live the best life possible.

Perhaps you've always had difficulties with self-esteem, and your illness only confirms your fears of inadequacy. If that's the case, you'll be distracted by false fears and unable to gain true insight into the actual deficits of your situation.

Exercise 16
Identification and Differentiation

Identification

1. List some fears, past and present, that have caused you to suffer.

2. Ask yourself these questions about each item

   When did you start having this fear?

   Why did/do you have this fear?

   Did something specific happen?

   Did pain or other physical symptoms occur?

   Did you become confused, disoriented?

   Did someone abandon you?

   Is there a specific person, place, or thing related to this fear?

   Other distinguishing features:

Differentiation

1. Do your fears, past and present, arise for the same reasons?

   If so, what are the reasons?

2. Do your fears arise for different reasons?

   If so, what are the reasons?

Try completing this exercise using losses or other causes of suffering.

Exercise 17
My Personality Characteristics

Describe what you were like before your illness.

Describe what you are like now.

What were your strengths in the past?

What are your strengths now?

What were your weaknesses in the past?

What are your weaknesses now?

What about your personality now most interferes with your changing your behavior?

What about your personality now most assists with your changing your behavior?

Maybe you're a perfectionist. You can't imagine how you can possibly stop doing any of your daily activities in the fashion that you've always done them. If you keep exhausting yourself into relapses, however, you've obviously got to find a new way to express orderliness in your life.

If you know that you have emotional problems in addition to your illness, or you suspect that perhaps your personality type or character is interfering with your learning how to live successfully with your illness, you should ask your medical team to refer you to a social worker, a psychologist, or a psychiatrist. These specialists can help you disentangle issues related to personality from those related to illness. They can also help you find ways to transform dysfunctional modes of behavior.

Completing Exercise 17, "My Personality Characteristics," may help you begin to think about who you are and how you can best learn to adapt to your present circumstances.

Assessing your hurts or traumas. You're very familiar with the physical hurts and injuries you've suffered because of your illness. And by now you're familiar with many of the emotional injuries as well. It's usually easy to identify physical injuries, but emotional ones are sometimes more difficult to identify. Some people have clear indicators that they're suffering trauma—they cry more than usual, or they have symptoms that concern or frighten them. Sometimes those around you become concerned about ways that you're behaving or symptoms you're having. But sometimes there aren't any clear indicators of trauma. If you have any doubts whatsoever about whether hurts you're suffering are serious or not, see your team for help immediately. If significant others in your life become concerned about your behavior or your symptoms, you should also see your health-care team. If you have serious traumas of any sort, you must go to your health-care team for help.

Phase two is the time for you to consider other ways that you've been hurt that you may not have considered. You still aren't the way you used to be. How are your friends, family, and co-workers reacting to you now? Do they consciously or unconsciously do or say things that give you pain? Perhaps they're withdrawing from you because they're emotionally overwhelmed or don't know what to do. This can still be traumatic for you, even if they aren't intentionally causing you pain.

How do your doctors treat you? Do they believe what you report to them? Do they listen to you? Are they getting frustrated because you're not responding better to treatment? You also need to think about how our culture at large regards your illness. Are you embarrassed or frightened to say that you're sick with your illness because you know that a recent TV program said it was all psychological? Exercise 18, "Assessing My Traumas," gives you space to write out these reactions so that you can examine them more clearly. Remember, you're looking here at physical and emotional hurts, injuries, and traumas.

Many people will tell you to emphasize the positive and not to dwell on pain or hurts that you've suffered. But you can't even hope to relieve a pain

Exercise 18
Assessing My Traumas

1. List some of your hurts, injuries, and traumas and where they occurred (home, social setting, doctor's office, workplace).

Physical	Occurred where	Emotional	Occurred where

2. About each one, consider the following.

   Was it caused by an individual?

   Was it caused by a group of people?

   How did it manifest itself?

   Was it caused by media or other general cultural stigmatization?

   If so, describe what happened.

3. Describe your feelings, thoughts, and behavior in reaction to each instance of hurt, injury, or trauma.

4. In a similar situation in the future, what would you do the same in terms of feelings, thoughts, and behavior?

5. In a similar situation, what would you do differently in terms of feelings, thoughts, and behavior?

unless you know about it. Your suffering will affect your life however you choose to deal with it, and I believe that you'll be much better off if you deal with it openly and consciously. In the coping and comfort section of this chapter I'll explore this further.

Maintaining insight. One of the hardest things to do in the world is to maintain insight. You can finally come to the realization that you push people away when you fear they may leave you, only to have this insight disappear completely the next time you fear someone's going to leave you. Even if you come to see that some of your expectations for yourself are totally unrealistic and you believe you've altered your ways, once you're back in your ordinary life it's hard not to revert to old ways and bad attitudes. After all, most people out in the world would prefer that you went back to being the person you used to be—you'd probably prefer it, too—and the society as a whole prefers totally healthy, young people. Everything can seem to conspire to dissolve any hard-won insight about living with chronic illness.

Exercise 19, "Insight Maintenance," will help you identify ways that you may lose insight and will help you increase your internal support for insight maintenance.

Values clarification and norm development. As you restructure the activities of your life, using the insight your observing self has developed, you'll automatically be developing new norms for your life. You want to consciously make clear to yourself what values you're asserting. Remember, by selecting one activity over another as you restructure your daily life, you're making a personal statement of what's important to you. You'll want to understand how you're making these judgments. This understanding is important because you'll want and need to share some of these values with the significant people in your life, both those who support you and help you maintain insight and those who encourage you to deny your insights. Completing Exercise 20, "Values Clarification and Norm Development," will help you see these issues more clearly. Use the exercise as a guide to write on separate sheets of paper, giving yourself as much room as you need to examine each questions completely.

Working with the Reactions of Others

Failure to return to the old you. As I mentioned earlier, the significant people in your life have begun to realize that you're not returning to the person you used to be. You're not "getting better." This creates a number of problems they didn't anticipate. Some of them just don't want to deal with the issue anymore. Others struggle to be helpful and behave well because they care about you a lot. But they may be hampered by a lack of understanding about what they should do or by an inability to take on any more obligations or activities in regard to you even though they wish they could.

Exercise 19
Insight Maintenance

Slips, Denial, and Self-Sabotage

1. List occasions when your insight is liable to slip.

Do they usually occur with certain people? If so, who?

Do they usually occur at certain places? If so, where?

Do they usually occur at certain times? If so, when?

2. List additional persons, places, and things or situations that tend to make you lose insight.

Examples: My close friend wants to do the things we used to.
Thanksgiving dinner is less stressful if I do the things I've always done.

3. Write down some of the reasons why you deny you're sick or limited.

Examples: Thinking about the truth makes me too sad.
Other people make it hard to keep the truth in mind.

4. Write down some of your denial statements.

Examples: They'll hate me if I cancel again.
I can do just one more household task, and then I'll rest.

5. List some of the ways that you begin sabotaging your own well-being.
Examples: I do the breakfast dishes because I just don't want to see them when I get home from work.

I'll visit my uncle this weekend because I don't want to have to explain yet again why visiting exhausts me.

Maintenance

1. List some of the people who help you maintain insight.
Examples: My social worker.

My new friend with MS.

2. List some of the places where you can best maintain insight.
Examples: At home in my bunker.

At the social worker's office.

3. List some of the occasions or things which help you maintain insight.
Examples: Listening to music tapes.

Sitting in the park at the duck pond.

4. List several reasons why you want to maintain your insight.
Examples: I want to feel better.

I want to lead a fuller life.

5. Write down some helpful maintenance statements
Examples: I am a good person.

I am a person worth loving just as I am.

Exercise 20
Values Clarification and Norm Development

1. What things are most important to you in your life? List in order of importance.

2. Reexamine your list.
   Do you personally value the items on your list, or are they things you believe you're supposed to value?

   Think about what you really value compared with what you are able to do. Taking your limitations into consideration, revise your values list.

3. List the activities in your life that support or promote each item on your revised values list. Include the amount of time you spend on each activity.

4. Compare your revised list of values with your list of activities that support your values.
   Do you spend most of your energy supporting the things you most value?

   Do you include activities from each of the four activity groups?

   Do you spend a lot of time and energy on activities unrelated to your revised values list?

5. Now create a new daily activities schedule which matches your values better and doesn't exhaust you (use Exercise 7).

Changed reactions. Consider how your friends, family, and co-workers are reacting to you now that it's apparent you're going to have your illness for a long time. You may want to fill out Exercises 9 through 13 again to see whether you would answer any of the questions differently now.

Phase two is often the most difficult period of chronic illness with regard to significant others. Old friendships, marriages, and families can all be disrupted, even permanently, because the individuals can't adjust to the complete change of life that your chronic illness may require. If you find that support, understanding, and sympathy for you is diminishing whether at home or in the workplace; you should immediately contact your counselor. This person can provide interventions with the other people in your life that may help them to understand and adapt. It is a sad truth, however, that some of your old relationships will probably not survive. But at the same time, you will be seeking out new people who support you, and integrating them into your life.

Roles and responsibilities. One reason relationships become so strained in phase two is that you and those around you have to revise your roles and responsibilities completely. You can't do all the things that you used to as a partner, a friend, a parent, or a worker. If you're married and you and your spouse have had busy lives with many activities, your partner may feel resentful and exhausted by the extra work your illness creates. This isn't what he or she signed up for. Your friends may not know how to have a relationship with you now since you can't do the things together that you used to. Your children may feel neglected, unloved, and scared by what seems to be happening to you. And your co-workers may feel that you're not pulling your weight.

Vicarious trauma. The other people in your life may be suffering what's called vicarious trauma. What's happening to you hurts them because it changes how you can be in relation to them. It also changes many other things about their lives. They've often got to take on jobs that you used to do. There may be financial stress because you're no longer able to work. Their suffering is just as real as yours. It needs to be acknowledged and addressed in the same way your traumas do. Your counselor can help you work with your family or the friends you live with both to acknowledge and grieve for their losses and to rearrange roles and responsibilities.

"Reducing keystrokes." You can often save considerable energy if you and your partner start reducing keystrokes. By this I mean that you do some life-maintenance jobs (the ADLs) less frequently and less intensely. It's not enough that you may have decided it's sufficient to clean your apartment only once a month. Your partner has to feel truly comfortable with this as well. Maybe you'll change the bed linen every other week or every third week. Maybe you'll buy more towels and underwear and do laundry only once a month. The important thing is that you and your significant others talk about what you're going to do. It's important that you all agree on decisions, and that you reach them together.

Values clarification and norm development. Just as you personally have to clarify your values as you restructure your daily activities, you and your family or friends together have to clarify the values that inform your relationship. Some people in your life may find it impossible to adjust to living with you as you are now. As hard as it may be, you'll most likely have to separate from these people. But most people who care about you want to try to understand. They, too, want to make a workable life with you. To do this, you and they need to talk about what values are most important in your lives together. You've got to be candid about what you can do and what you need. But you've also got to recognize that they probably won't be able to pick up all the slack so that your life together runs just about the way it used to. Together you can talk about how to reduce the keystrokes of necessary activities, but you also have to recognize that your entire life together will have to change. You'll almost certainly have to eliminate some activities and streamline others. But this becomes possible if together you have worked out what your essential values are. With your significant others, complete Exercise 21, "Household Values Clarification and Norm Development" on separate sheets of paper.

Financial issues. One of the biggest changes chronic illness produces involves your finances. These altered circumstances can be very frightening and stress-provoking. Many people with chronic illness must either cut back to part-time work or must cease working altogether. As a household, you almost certainly will be living with less income than you used to have. Some people with chronic illness are able to get disability, which may help, but it rarely makes up the difference of your lost salary. Your counselor can help work with you regarding financial issues.

The first thing you or you and your partner need to do is work up an actual budget that shows you exactly what income you have and how much you're spending now. Some chronically ill people find that although they lose income, they also cease spending money on certain things like evenings out or ski trips, because they can't do these things any longer. In addition to your counselor, you and your partner may want to talk with a financial advisor about your best strategies for making the most of your income. Exercise 22, "Financial Issues," will help you review the issue of your finances.

Illness etiquette. You and your family need to learn how to behave around others regarding your illness. You need to know what to say, how to say it, to whom, and when. Maybe it's necessary for you to say something to your boss, or an in-law, or a well-meaning but hurtful friend. You have to explain about your illness and what you can and can't do now. Don't just wing it. Figure out what points you want to make. Then write out the conversation and practice speaking it. As you do this, you'll diffuse some of the raw emotion that you may have been feeling as you first thought about the conversation—the anger or fear or annoyance—and you can get to a place where you make your statements calmly and reasonably.

Exercise 21
Household Values Clarification
and Norm Development

1. Each family member should complete Exercise 20. An adult should help any children in the family to answer the questions.

2. Using your separate lists, discuss with your partner or family members the things that are most important to both or all of you in your life. Create a combined list, putting items in order of importance.

3. Discuss and list below what activities are necessary to support these values. Make sure to consider activities from each of the four activity groups. Remember to include the reduction of keystrokes in performing family ADLs.

4. Discuss which person will perform each activity.
   Will it actually be possible for the person to do this job?

   If the person is you, will you have enough energy or strength, given the other activities you must accomplish each day?

   If the person is not you, will that person have time do to this job in addition to his or her other activities? Will the person have the capacity to do the job? (Children are sometimes not old enough to take on certain activities. Elderly family members may not have the strength or energy either.)

5. Are you able to assign all the activities necessary to support your household values or do you need to rethink what values you can and wish to support?

6. If you revise your household values, set up a new schedule of activities for each household member.

Exercise 22
Financial Issues

1. List your total household income by source.

Source	Amount	Total
		_____

2. If you will be leaving your job or cutting down to part-time work, reduce your income by that amount and write your new total on this line.

_____

3. List your total household expenses. Check whether each is an Obligation (such as taxes, mortgage, insurance, etc.), a Variable (food, clothing, etc.), or Optional (entertainment, vacations, etc.)

Item	Obligation	Variable	Optional	Amount	Total

4. Compare your expenses to your revised total income. If your expenses exceed your income, you'll need to do some budget planning.
   It is **not** advisable simply to eliminate optional items because they can make a great difference in your quality of life. You must budget for activities in all four activity groups.

   You need to consider the entire picture, including how your activities have changed now that you're ill. If you've taken expense figures from before you were ill, reexamine them. Certain expense figures will probably have changed.

You may wish to consult with a financial planner. Many issues are involved in your financial picture, such as tax changes, for which you may need professional advice.

You may need to confront a health-care provider about behavior you find unsatisfactory. The power distribution between patient and doctor in our culture can make it very difficult for you as a patient to question your doctor's decisions, analysis, or behavior. But your illness doesn't reduce your value as a human being or your right to courteous, professional treatment. If you have difficulty developing "scripts" for talking with people about your illness, enlist the aid of your counselor. Having a real person to generate ideas and practice with can help get rid of your understandable "stage fright."

Work and disability. If you're still able to work, issues at your job often come to a head during phase two. Most jobs can absorb short periods of illness in any employee. But if the illness or absences persist, then your employer and co-workers begin to want changes. Employers sometimes want to fire employees who can't perform to the level they want. But many employers must comply with the Americans with Disabilities Act. If you've got a disability—and many of the problems of chronic illness qualify as disabilities—many employers have to make accommodations to your needs.

If you've been sick a long time, your co-workers probably don't want to take on your work as a regular thing. Also, they may be scared by your illness.

Your counselor can be of invaluable help in this area. He or she can bring in a physical or occupational therapist to suggest ergonomic modifications at your workstation so that you can do your job with less strain and more efficient expenditure of energy. The counselor can speak with your employer or your co-workers about the nature of your illness, thus letting these people know what you can do and why they don't need to fear you. It's possible that your job can be modified or you can work part-time.

Or you may need to stop work altogether, at least for a while. Your counselor can work with you and your medical team to help prepare your disability case. This is not easy to do. You need to have the advice of someone well-versed in the pitfalls and problems of applying for disability.

Comfort and Coping

"The enforced monastic life." In phase two you're able to come out of the bunker of phase one, but you still have to live a very contained, attentive life for a while. This is what I mean by the enforced monastic life. As you examine and restructure your life activities, you need to pay very close attention. In phase one you tried to reduce your activities to the most essential ADLs, and even those you tried to streamline. As you do your ADLs now, think about each process. Think about the fact that you're accomplishing necessary work. You need to begin to honor all the actions you take and to see value in them, even if they're as humble as getting up and shaving every morning.

As you begin to restructure your activities in the other three categories, you want to pay close attention to each one that you are thinking about including in your new life. What do you do in this activity? Can you do it in a more efficient way? Is this activity one that means a lot to you? You want to develop a conscious awareness of every action. What is it? How is it done? What does it mean to you? Consciously honoring your activities is an essential element in the enforced monastic existence.

Structure is also an important component, which is why I call the life "monastic." You carefully choose a limited number of activities and add them slowly and deliberately to your new life. Structure is important right now because your old world has been turned completely upside down. None of your old reference points are reliable anymore. You're a little like a kid who's just learning how to walk. You don't know where you can go, and you tend to lurch off in any direction. As a kid, your parents provided a safe area for you to experiment with this new skill of walking. They set safe boundaries. That's what you're doing for yourself now. You're setting up close, safe boundaries of action for you in your new situation.

It's hard to believe now, but these little steps are going to lead you eventually to a meaningful and fulfilling life.

Expanding relationships and comfort zones. Now that you've entered phase two, you can actually emerge from the bunker of phase one. You've probably already begun to reach out to meet people who will be supportive and understanding. Having set up a safe, restful place at home and reduced your required actions to the minimum, you can now begin to add other activities to your life. But you must consider thoughtfully what's important to make part of your new life and what from your old life you're going to discard, at least for now.

Engaging your grief reaction. With the greater calm and energy capacity of phase two, you need to consciously engage your grief reaction. You've experienced, and will continue to experience, suffering and loss. You need to be aware of this so that your suffering finds conscious expression, rather than emerging unbidden in destructive or embarrassing ways. Even the true advance from bunker to enforced monastic living may seem like a huge loss when you think about your old life.

You've got to allow yourself to feel and then express as emotively as possible the sadness or the fury and the loss. Make some time during the day when you can be private and simply feel whatever your feelings are. Cry if you want. Express your anger or rage. Find a place (like in your car on a quiet road with the windows rolled up) where you can scream or yell out all the things that enrage you. Use felt-tipped markers to make a big, bold list of everything that makes you angry. Sometimes listening to music or writing in a journal helps open you to your feelings of loss and suffering. It doesn't matter how you bring it about. It may even happen accidentally sometimes as you're performing tasks that once were simple and now require great attention and effort on your part. You can't depend on accidental moments, however. You've got to make special time for what is really an important activity of daily life and personal fulfillment. What's important is allowing and expressing the feelings at a time and a place that you choose.

When you try to be stoic about your suffering, or think only positive thoughts, you expend a lot of energy suppressing your feelings. You hide your grief from your conscious attention. But your grief and loss haven't gone away. They will find a way out. If you don't make time to express your grief and loss, they'll make their own time. You're apt to burst into tears at undesirable moments, such as when you're at the grocery store or in a social gathering. Or else you may find yourself furiously berating your partner for not putting the car in the garage. But you're really getting angry because of the rage you feel at what's happened to you. These feelings have to find expression somewhere.

If you don't attend to your suffering consciously, you'll suffer neurotically and make yourself and others miserable. Making others miserable pushes them away. This will make you even more miserable and deprive you of the support and good will that's absolutely essential to you. You become more and more isolated and irritable.

Meeting your suffering with compassion. In phase one you were encouraged to *allow* your suffering, to acknowledge that it's there. In phase two I encourage you to express your grief about your suffering, but also to regard your suffering with *compassion*. You've been forced to experience pain and loss, but you shouldn't punish yourself for this. On the contrary, you need to try feeling compassion for yourself as you would for the suffering of another.

Structured spiritual support. While you may have felt spiritually abandoned in the crisis phase, in phase two you may find some comfort and support in the structured spiritual practices of the religion you grew up in. This may be the first time that the beliefs you were taught as a child have ever been subject to a real test. Perhaps you're anxious to see whether the practices of prayer and service attendance will help you.

Or maybe you've been long distanced from the faith of your childhood. You may now be seeking something that will help sustain you in this time of trouble. Perhaps you've become attracted to the sources of spiritual support that have helped the new friends you've made who have your illness. If those people who know the kind of suffering and loss you've experienced can find comfort and help in a particular spiritual practice, perhaps you think it will work for you as well.

Regular attendance at services, regular prayer, and regular meditation can all contribute powerfully to supporting you as you try to restructure your life.

Moving Toward Resolution

In phase two your goal is to stabilize and begin restructuring your life. You do this by living an enforced monastic life in which you pay close attention to all your activities. You think carefully as you begin to define the boundaries of your new life and as you select activities from the four general categories to include in that life. Psychologically you use your personal narrative to develop your skills of self-observation. You analyze your current situation and attempt to maintain the insights you gain. You attempt to go beyond your psychological defenses so that you can move forward to the process of developing new norms and clarifying your values. With the significant people in your life, you attempt to deal with the problems that arise because your illness is chronic, and you're probably not going to return to "normal." This means openly addressing issues of roles and responsibilities, finances, and values clarification. Both at home and at work you may find your counselor can provide interventions that help to resolve difficult situations. You make time to grieve for your suffering and losses, and you regard your suffering with compassion.

You're now entering phase three, the resolution phase, which I'll discuss in the next chapter. You've come to understand deeply that your condition is chronic and that you'll never return to your pre-crisis self. But at the same time, you've learned many coping skills that make your life more manageable and richer. Because you've got greater awareness of social stigmatization and are working to build your network of positive supporters, you've got higher self-esteem. In phase three you'll start learning to become your own health-care advocate and activities monitor. You'll develop ongoing methods for keeping your family, friends, and work life on track. And you'll begin to construct the new, authentic you. This new self encompasses much of your pre-crisis self, but much more besides. Most importantly, in phase three you'll be committing yourself to the all-important issue of developing a deep, personal sense of meaning. Difficult though this task is, you'll learn how to approach it through a variety of sustaining, fulfilling creative actions. Throughout these efforts, authenticity will be the ultimate measure of personal attitudes, friendships, and all issues of meaning.

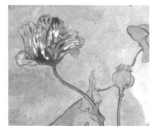

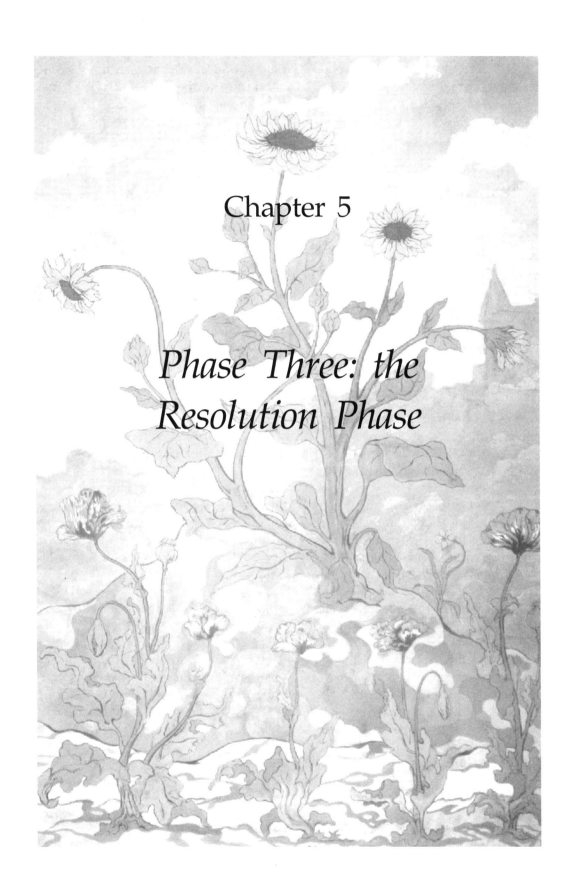

Chapter 5

Phase Three: the Resolution Phase

During phase two you stabilized your new situation of living with a chronic illness. Gradually you began adding to the bare minimum of activities that you carried out during phase one. You have continued to take care not to exceed your energy levels. When you find that you are doing too much, you cut back again. In the process, you have begun constructing a new life, one that includes activities from all four categories. As you have accomplished these things, you have also moved toward phase three, the resolution phase. What are the signs that you've actually entered phase three?

Resolution

You know your condition is chronic. One of the most important indicators that you're entering phase three is your profound recognition that you have a chronic illness. You now know in your heart of hearts that you're not going to be cured, at least not in any foreseeable future. You're never going to return to life as it used to be before you got sick.

For many people in phase two, their physical plateau or their familiarity with their regular symptoms makes them hope that they are actually getting better. So it's not unusual for people to get stuck in a cycle where they think they're getting better, they attempt to return to their old life, they overdo, and they suffer a severe relapse that returns them to a phase one crisis state. Gradually they contain the crisis and begin to stabilize into phase two again. Eventually, however, their symptom regularity again convinces them that they're "better," and they push themselves into crisis again. This cycle can repeat over and over again when chronically ill people refuse to recognize that their condition is for all practical purposes permanent. But if you have carried out the self-examination activities of phase two thoughtfully, you've almost assuredly come to recognize that your condition is chronic—that is, you'll most likely live with it permanently.

You've got a greater and greater sense of control over your situation. There are deep difficulties associated with acknowledging that your condition is chronic. I'll get to them in this chapter. But one advantage of this recognition is that you've simultaneously acquired a deep sense that you can find help and improvement in yourself. It doesn't all depend on your doctor or counselor, even though these people are extremely important in helping you. Better living comes from within yourself. Much of it depends on how you behave and what you choose to do.

You've learned to differentiate your responses. In phase three you don't assume that everything that happens to you occurs because of your illness. You recognize that people sometimes behave toward you in annoying or hurtful ways for reasons that have nothing to do with your illness. You also recognize that you may feel sad or anxious or pressured to act in certain ways not just because of your illness but sometimes because of how you've always reacted to certain kinds of situations in your life. Sometimes it's because of the illness, but sometimes it's not.

You're increasingly aware of society's stigmatization. You can now see pretty clearly that society's attitudes can create a lot of the difficulties you encounter. This is a problem that I'll talk about below, but at least you no longer agree with this social attitude. You don't think it expresses something true. Most of the time you don't blame yourself for your illness, and you don't think you're bad, or mad, or malingering.

You've got higher self-esteem. Because you're more conscious of how you can be stigmatized by society's attitudes, your self-esteem is greater. You don't feel that you're at fault, so you refuse to think badly of yourself because of your illness. On the contrary, you may actually be developing a degree of admiration for how well you're handling your new situation. You've also probably found other people with your condition, and their support and understanding has helped to rebuild your self-esteem.

You're better able to live with the ambiguity and chronic nature of your condition. While you don't like being ill, you're a lot more used to your condition than you were at the start. You know now that it's always hard to say what any tomorrow is going to be like. Your situation is ambiguous. You may be relatively fine for months, only to suffer renewed symptoms or altogether new ones. You may have come to recognize patterns in your symptoms, or triggers that set off periods of increased symptoms. But you know that the symptoms of your illness can and probably will change at any time in the future.

You openly express compassion for yourself. You don't always try to hide from yourself or others that you've suffered a lot and continue to suffer because of your illness. You recognize that it's important for you to allow yourself to acknowledge your suffering. You know that you must also feel compassion for yourself. You've had losses and continue to have losses—some chronically ill people suffer tremendous losses—and you need to respond compassionately to yourself and your suffering.

You're consciously constructing a story of your illness experience. Early on you began to try to tell the story of what has happened to you. As you moved through phase two, you examined your illness narrative much more critically, separating out issues that were related to your illness from issues that weren't. In phase three you'll apply even deeper thought to your story, because now you're doing it in full consciousness that your illness is chronic. You no longer secretly believe that the next doctor, guru, or medication will "cure" you, returning life to the way it used to be.

Strategy: Finding Meaning in the Tunnel

Goal. The goal in phase three is to develop meaning and to construct a new self. I call the strategy for doing this "finding meaning in the tunnel." You know the expression of seeing the light at the end of the tunnel? It tells you that despite the dark and difficult times you may be going through, you suddenly see a light that promises you that you'll soon escape from your present difficulties into a wonderful, bright, happy place.

I'm not going to promise you that. As you enter phase three and recognize deeply that your situation is permanent, you'll probably feel great despair. You may feel like you're trapped in a tunnel of darkness and hopelessness. Chronic illness will not let you escape from the permanence of your situation, but you can discover meaning while you're in that dreary tunnel. You can come to honor what you do while you're there. And this—you may have to take it on faith from me right now—will ultimately change your life. You'll cease to be in the tunnel, even if you're not in a place of bright bliss.

As in the previous phases, you're going to accomplish this strategy through tactics and skills aimed at your physical self, your psychological self, and yourself as you relate to others.

Assuming management of your physical care. If you are physically and mentally capable, part of your phase three sense of control and competence allows you to put yourself firmly in charge of your physical well-being. You become your own care coordinator, health-care advocate, and activity monitor.

Acting creatively to develop meaning. Psychologically you've arrived at a point where you must engage the big existential questions. Why did this happen to me? Why am I here? What possible meaning can my life have now? You'll move toward answering these questions by engaging in creative activity that will in turn help you to develop a very personal, authentic sense of the meaning of your life.

Taking control in your wider world. You and those around you both now recognize that you're chronically ill. This means that your life and theirs must change permanently. During the activities of phase two, you and your significant others began grappling with the important issues of living with illness. In phase three, you work together with them to set up ongoing ways to evaluate and reevaluate issues of role, responsibility, interaction, companionship, work relations, and so forth. You also continue to build new friendships and relationships with supporters whom you began to find during phase two.

In this phase, even more than the earlier two phases, you'll be completing the exercises several times. You'll also sometimes be asking others to work with you on this or to fill out similar forms themselves. So you'll need to make several copies of each exercise form so that you'll be able to fill out a clean form several different times.

Tactics and Skills

Assuming Management of Your Physical Care

Your long-term symptom status. By phase three you've learned that you can experience almost any symptom status. You may have long periods of plateau in which your symptoms remain more or less the same. Or they may change in cycles that you recognize and feel you can manage. You may even experience symptom improvement. But you also know that you can have relapses. These relapses may be totally unrelated to anything you've done— they just happen. Some people have chronic illnesses with a known downward progression. If your condition is one of these, this is also something you'll be aware of by now.

As a reminder to yourself of the general picture of your symptoms, complete Exercise 23, "A General Overview of My Symptom Pattern." You'll want to adjust the exercise so that the symptoms correspond with your particular illness, just as you did in Exercise 5. Using the scale of 1 to 5 that you used in that exercise, write in the box for each symptom in Exercise 23 how severe that symptom generally was or is now for the time period you're filling out. Remember, your symptoms will not necessarily bear a relation to the phase you're in. Symptoms are manifestations of your illness. The phase you're in indicates your level of coping.

You become your own care coordinator. If you developed the sort of medical team in phase one that I recommended, your team leader assumed most of the tasks of your physical care coordination during phase one and two. This person kept track of all your clinicians, medications, and other protocols. The team leader kept all parties informed about the treatments other clinicians ordered. This person also raised questions when one protocol or medication seemed to contradict or work poorly with another.

Over the course of phase two, illness permitting, you started to learn how to do this yourself. You'll complete the process in phase three. You learn by observing and understanding what your team leader has done. You learn what to ask your doctors, what to tell them, and how to interpret the ways your particular, individual body reacts to different treatments. You learn when symptom changes require that you check in with your doctors immediately rather than waiting for regular checkups. By the end of phase three you're ready to assume control. This doesn't mean that you never call on your team leader. It's just that you don't need this person's help and advice as much as you did in the past.

Complete Exercise 24, "Reporting to My Medical Team," along with your health-care team leader. The form of Exercise 24 in this book is actually an example to give you and your health-care team a framework in which to develop your own, individualized exercise. You and your team leader need to select your own red-flag items, your own symptoms to report in twenty-four and forty-eight hours, etc., so that the items fit your illness and your

Exercise 23
A General Overview of My Symptom Pattern

Remember: Your physical symptoms occur independently of the phase you are in. You may never have experienced a relapse after you reach a plateau of symptoms. Some individuals experience many relapses and improvements. Others do not.

Directions: Refer to Exercise 5. Adjust the symptoms to fit your illness. Use the symptom severity scale of 1 to 5 that you used in Exercise 5. This time, however, assess your overall symptom severity during each period of time (onset, plateau 1, etc.).

	Fatigue	Cognitive	Headache	Sore Throat	Body Ache	GI Problems	Anxiety	Depression
Original Crisis								
Plateau 1								
Relapse/ Improvement 1								
Plateau 2								
Relapse/ Improvement 2								
Plateau 3								

doctor's recommendations. When you and your team leader have constructed an Exercise 24 appropriate to you, you should then review it with your doctor. After you have adjusted the items in accordance with your doctor's suggestions, ask the doctor to sign the exercise to indicate that he or she agrees that those are the correct procedures for you to follow.

You become your own health advocate. You also learn, starting with the work you began in phase two, to recognize whether you're receiving the kind of health care you have a right to expect. If you're not, you are learning how to correct the situation. Moreover, the growth of your self-esteem and your development of supporters help empower you to act and enable you to speak for yourself and your legitimate expectations. In phase three you usually recognize stigmatization when it occurs, and you understand the subtle ways in which you can suffer iatrogenic trauma. You no longer suffer these kinds of hurts or trauma without comment because you're afraid of alienating the clinician. Instead you stand up for yourself and insist on being treated professionally. If you're not, you find a new provider.

You become your own activities monitor. In phase three you no longer struggle to "pass" for normal because you recognize that your condition is chronic and that passing behavior worsens your situation. You're therefore far less likely to overdo your activities. You may try to include in your life as much as you physically can, but you recognize limits and impose them on yourself when you're tired or depleted. You know that you need to examine your activity level periodically to make sure that you're living within sustainable boundaries. Because you have greater self-esteem, you trust your judgment more. This is not to say that good friends or the person whom you selected earlier as your activities monitor won't alert you when they think you're pushing your limits. And you listen to them. But you've internalized the need to act wisely, so you have less need to rely on outside advice.

Complete Exercise 25, "My Activities Assessment." You'll probably want to do it several times. You may want it to reflect a day's activities for a while, and then a week's activities. In this exercise, pay particular attention to your distribution of activities over the four activity areas. Notice the activities where you tend to overdo and make reminder notes to yourself ahead of such occasions. If possible, try to spell out how you can do this activity less intensely. If you know that you'll carry out the activity the way you always have, then make specific plans to reduce other activities afterwards so that you can recover.

Static vs. dynamic disability. In phase three you learn the nature of disability. Most people tend to regard disability as a static, unchanging, visible thing. Maybe you used to think that way, too. Most people think a disabled person is someone in a wheelchair or someone being guided by a Seeing Eye dog. Some people do have static disabilities, although many of them are actually invisible to outside observers.

Exercise 24
Reporting to My Medical Team

Directions: Create a medical report system with your health-care team leader, using the form below as a model. When you have completed it, have your doctor review it, make any necessary alterations, and sign it as an indication that these are the reporting procedures you should follow.

Red Flag Items

Report these matters immediately! If you cannot reach your doctor, call the contact you designated for medical emergencies in Exercise 2.

Example: Drug reactions (fever, rash, swelling, choking, breathing difficulties); Pay particular attention if you're just beginning a new prescription medication, over-the-counter drug, or herbal or nutritional supplement.

Report within Twenty-four Hours

Examples: Fever
Dizziness, loss of balance
Sudden pain or dramatic increase of familiar pain
Vomiting

Report within Forty-eight Hours

Examples: Significant alteration in habitual symptoms
Appearance of new symptoms
Persistent low fever

Report at 6-Month/Annual Checkups

Examples: Report status of your habitual symptoms (see Exercise 23), noting fluctuations;
Ask doctor about questions and concerns since last visit (make list).

Approved by doctor _____

Exercise 25
My Activities Assessment

Directions: List your activities in each time period. Indicate the activity group (ADL, personal fulfillment, social, work) the activity is in. Estimate the time spent on each task. Assess your energy expenditure on each task. Review Exercise 3 and Exercise 14 when completing this exercise.

Do this exercise over an extended period of time. Try filling in items in the morning, in the afternoon, and in the evening. Examine the exercise when you're feeling relatively full of energy and when you're tired. Fill it in several times and compare your copies.

	Activity and Activity Group	Amount of Time	Okay/ Overdoing
Morning at home/work			
Noon/ lunchtime			
Afternoon at home/work			
Dinnertime			
Evening			

Exercise 26
My Disabilities

1. List your disabilities under the appropriate categories, either "Dynamic" or "Static." Briefly describe the nature of each disability and its range in the dynamic category.

Dynamic	Static
Physical	Physical
Cognitive	Cognitive
Sleep	Others?
Digestion	
Capacity to drive	
Others?	

2. List equipment you need when you're experiencing greater disability.

Disability	Equipment

The great majority of chronically ill people have disabilities that are dynamic. You're more or less disabled depending on the particular symptoms you're experiencing at any particular time and their severity. Disability for many chronically ill people is invisible because it takes the form of continuous pain or debilitating fatigue. But whether your disabling symptoms are visible or not, you are still disabled during that period of time. You should use all the services and provisions made available by law to anyone with a disability.

Complete Exercise 26, "My Disabilities." Fill out the two columns, one each for static and dynamic disabilities. Most of your problems probably fall in the dynamic category. Try to identify any triggering conditions that increase your disabilities so that you can be mindful of them. If triggering situations are unavoidable, you can still prepare to ease the experience by having the proper equipment available (wheelchairs, disability parking permits, etc.).

Acting Creatively to Develop Meaning

Revisiting your personal narrative. Regularly throughout the phase process you should reexamine your personal narrative, particularly as it relates to your illness. You can be gaining insight all the time about yourself, those close to you, your health-care providers, your co-workers, and society at large. As a consequence, it's helpful to review and edit your original interpretations of experience to see if your judgment was clouded by things you didn't see or understand when you first told your story. You also want to add information about what has happened since you began the narrative.

You're trying to give the most authentic, truthful account of your life that you can. During the construction of your new self during phase three, you're going to use only those things that are genuinely, authentically what you think, feel, and believe. Your story helps to guide you toward these true aspects of yourself.

Deep mourning for your lost self. When you finally recognize that you've got a chronic—a permanent—illness, it throws into stark relief everything that you've lost. You now must consciously acknowledge that your old life is never coming back. You can't perform your old roles in the way you used to. Your partner may have left you because she or he can't adjust to your changed life. If you've got children, they may be confused, perhaps even scared of the person you seem to have become. You've doubtless lost some old friends who used to mean the world to you. You've assuredly lost many of your old activities, to say nothing of your sense of vibrancy and vitality. You've often lost your old personality. These are huge losses, and it's urgent in phase three that you grieve for them. You can't move forward if you don't express the intense feelings that so much loss occasions. Many people find it helps to work with a professional to identify their losses and mourn them appropriately.

Complete Exercise 27, "My Losses, External and Internal." Try to do this exercise, and several of the exercises that follow, slowly over a period of time.

You'll also benefit by talking about it with others like your partner, your friends, and your counselor. You want to capture how you feel both when you're feeling good, but also when you're feeling tired and discouraged. Consider the questions in this exercise at your most active times of the day, but also at the times when you're most exhausted. You don't have to list absolutely everything here, but you should try to identify what losses affect you most deeply. You need to name them consciously and intentionally so that you can grieve for them properly.

Existential questions loom. When your old self dies, and your old life ends, of course you're going to experience great dread and confusion. Who am I now? you ask. Why should I live? How should I live? Why did this happen to me? Why do bad things happen to anyone? What kind of universe is this? At the beginning of phase three, chronically ill individuals often feel like they've fallen into a dark pit. They're in the depths of despair.

Dark night of the soul. Some people call this deep existential despair the "dark night of the soul." Others say it's just depression. Actually, it's usually both. If you're feeling desperate or suicidal, you should immediately seek medical help. It may be recommended or you may choose to use medications that will calm and settle you so that you'll be able to process the material that will allow you to travel through your existential dark night.

It's important to remember that you're not simply feeling depressed. You're also asking vitally important, soul-shaking questions that all people should ask themselves. Most people don't, however, until life throws something horrendous in their way. In the process of answering these questions, you're going to discover what is deeply true and meaningful for you. This meaning may or may not resemble what religious or secular authorities say is meaningful—it's more about what *you* find true, deep within yourself.

Phoenix from the ashes. Perhaps you've heard the myth of the phoenix, a bird that lives 500 years and then burns itself up in a fire, only to reemerge out of the flames completely renewed for another 500 years. This is what's going to happen to you. You're going to emerge from the dark night, the tunnel—whatever metaphoric image you want—as a new self, as a person who combines qualities from both your past self and your present explorations.

It's almost impossible for most people at the beginning of phase three to believe that they can ever get to a better place. This is why it may help you to find a good counselor to accompany you during your exploration. You'll probably need to borrow the faith of someone else at first. Find it in friends, in a counselor, in a support group, wherever, but don't stop looking until you find it. You can emerge from this difficult time. What follows are some of the ways that you do this.

Committing to time in the tunnel. First, you've got to commit yourself to spending time in the dark tunnel. Although everything may seem hopeless

Exercise 27
My Losses, External and Internal

Directions: Do this exercise over an extended period of time. Try filling in items in the morning, in the afternoon, and in the evening. Examine the exercise when you're feeling relatively full of energy and when you're tired. Fill it in several times and compare your copies. Discuss your losses with others—your partner, your friends, or counselor.

External Losses

Activity	Value for you	Is it totally lost?

Internal Losses

Characteristic or behavior	Value for you	Is it totally lost?

and pointless to you, you've got to commit to the effort of trying to make something out of this experience. Unless you deal with the issues of being and purpose, you'll probably find yourself slipping back into a repetitive phase one/phase two cycle because almost inevitably you'll retreat to the notion that somehow there's a way for you to return to your old life.

Maintaining insight and issue reframing. Once committed to the process of searching for meaning, you focus initially on maintaining the insights about life and relationships that you've gained as you analyzed your situation in phase two. This can be very difficult because your pain can be so great that you have difficulty maintaining your hard-won insights.

As a consequence, you've got to remember to keep reframing issues that come up. Reframing can sometimes seem as irritatingly simplistic as the statement "when life gives you lemons, make lemonade." But reframing is much more complicated and truthful than that. Reframing helps you transform your apparently tragic circumstances into heroic ones. This is not a pretend activity where you fool yourself. It's a matter of looking at your situation from a different viewpoint. It's about learning how to play the poor hand that life has dealt you in the best way possible. You go from being a passive victim to being an active hero.

To give you an example: One young woman was unable to complete high school because of the many difficulties relating to her illness. Eventually, however, after studying on her own, she insisted on taking college entrance exams. She passed them, went to college, and despite great difficulties, earned her bachelor's degree. This woman could view herself as a high school dropout. But she refused to accept that role. Instead, quite correctly, she regards her striving for and attainment of a college degree as a heroic quest demonstrating her true intrinsic value. Reframing issues helps you to maintain your new insights and keep from falling back into old, dysfunctional patterns.

Defining your pre-crisis self. You now begin to identify just who you used to be. You want to think in terms of your character and your personality, your activities, friendships, jobs, relationships—everything. Exercise 28, "My Pre-Crisis Self," will help you to list these things. This exercise is one to complete slowly, over many days. Consider the items privately, but you most definitely also want to talk about them with the other people in your life and with your counselor or illness support group friends. Try to think about the various categories at different times of the day, when you're feeling upbeat and when you're feeling tired or down. A true picture of your pre-crisis self will emerge if you consider it in all sorts of different situations and with the many different people who are important to you.

What is lost? Go down the list in Exercise 28 and compare with Exercise 27. For each defining item, think about whether this is something that you've lost. Perhaps, for example, you used to be an enthusiastic skier, but now you're suffering with severe rheumatoid arthritis. Because your physical disability won't permit you to ski anymore, this is an actual loss.

Exercise 28
My Pre-Crisis Self

Directions: Do this exercise over an extended period of time. Try filling in items in the morning, in the afternoon, and in the evening. Examine the exercise when you're feeling relatively full of energy and when you're tired. Fill it in several times and compare your copies. Discuss your pre-crisis self with others—your partner, your friends, your counselor.

Jot down as many characteristics about each category as you can think of. Ask yourself what you were like before your illness/disability in this area.

Character	
Personality	
Activities	
Friendships	
Social Life	
Job/Employment	

Perhaps you've listed that you're a parent. When you think about all the things you can't do with and for your children now, you think about loss. But have you actually lost the ability to be a parent? Or have you only lost the way that you used to be one? You may not be able to coach the soccer team or take your kids camping, but perhaps your relative inaction nowadays may make it possible to be a more attentive, listening parent. This is not a loss, but rather a defining quality for which you need to find new modes of expression.

Perhaps in the old days you used to join the phone banks for public radio fund-raising marathons. But you can't talk easily anymore because your Sjogren's syndrome interferes. It's true that you may not be able to support causes you care about in that way, but are you prevented from supporting them in other ways?

These are external things—things you do or relationships you have with other people. But perhaps you've suffered internal losses as well. These can be the hardest to take. Perhaps you used to be a confident, outgoing, authoritative person. Now you're cautious and unsure. Naturally you see this as a loss. You may not even particularly like the person you've become. But if you allow yourself to observe objectively, you may find that your new personality traits permit you to see some things with greater clarity. They may permit you to form new and rewarding relationships because you allow others to act.

In Exercise 29, "What Have I Actually Lost," consider what aspects of "lost" characteristics or activities are truly lost, and which ones you may be able to do in different ways. Again, try to do this exercise over a period of time, discussing the issues with others and thinking about them by yourself as well.

Finding baseline authenticity. Authenticity is the key to making your new self and your new life, but it can be very hard to achieve. It takes a lot of time and practice to get to an authentic life. You're going to make many false starts and stops. You'll need to "try on" a lot of things to see how you feel about them. But if you keep working at it, it gets easier.

Begin by looking at Exercise 28 again. Did you actually *like* doing all the things you listed? Some daily maintenance activities bore everyone, but we've got to do them. But did you enjoy the people you were involved with? Did you engage in some activities and relationships because it seemed necessary in terms of your job, or because your partner expected it of you, or because you just thought that's what all people do?

In Exercise 30, "Things That Are Authentically Me," write down things that you can do and relationships that you can have in your present situation that you really truly, deeply want. Choose things that *you* want, not the ones that you think you *should* want or that you think *others* think you should want. If you can, write down reasons why these relationships or these activities are essential to you. This is yet another exercise you want to complete over time and with the input of others. Ultimately, you alone will be the judge of what's truly "you." But how others see you and what they think is important to you can often make you see things that you have never really noticed about yourself. Sometimes your friends, your partner, or your counselor know parts of you better than you do because you've never really reflected on these things yourself before. It's also important to remember that items in the list in Exercise 30 and how you feel about them will change as time goes on.

As you construct your new self, make sure that you're not pretending about anything. You're going to make a lot of false starts and stops. That's normal. As I said before you'll need to try on all sorts of things. See if they might actually fit you. You may find new ways to be that never occurred to you in the past. Try hard to be absolutely honest with yourself and true to how you really feel. You'll be glad you did, because most chronically ill people experience extraordinary relief when they can stop pretending.

Experimenting with opposites. One way to help locate what you truly want and feel is to experiment in your imagination with completely antithetical roles, identities, or emotions. Imagine yourself as someone totally different from the person you used to be. If you've always been the leader, suggesting what everyone's going to do and making arrangements for events, imagine becoming very passive. Imagine letting others do the suggesting. Imagine letting them do all the arranging. See how you feel when you don't attempt to take charge, but simply go with the flow.

Perhaps you've always been a person who accommodates to the needs and wishes of others. You may never have developed very strong feelings about anything, so it's been easy for you to fit in with the strong preferences of those around you. Imagine doing the opposite. Try to think of choices you would make and how you would persuade others to go along with your preferences.

If you've always been a strong, stoic type, imagine expressing every emotion that comes into your head. Try complaining mentally about every annoyance and difficulty. Imagine telling everyone who helps you how important they are to you and how much you love them.

Activities such as these can give you an entirely different perspective on your old behavior. They may also give you insight into new ways you might prefer to adopt. Perhaps you took on certain roles or behaviors in the past because no one else would or because you thought it was expected of you. Now you not only *can* change, but you *must* change to fit with a self that's authentically you.

Engaging in creative activities. One of the best ways to discover your authentic self is to engage your creative processes. You've already begun working creatively with your issue reframing. Creative activity is personally rewarding. Furthermore, if the activity is truly rewarding to you, it draws out your most honest expressions of yourself. Some people like to write. Others prefer to paint or carve or play the guitar or sing or build things. Creativity may consist of tying fishing flies or training dogs or becoming involved in political activities. Cutting out magazine photos to make collages is creative work. Music is a wonderful creative activity, even if you're primarily a

Exercise 29
What Have I Actually Lost

Directions: Do this exercise over an extended period of time. Try completing items in the morning, in the afternoon, and in the evening. Examine the exercise when you're feeling relatively full of energy and when you're tired. Fill it in several times and compare your copies. Discuss what you have actually lost with others—your partner, your friends, your counselor.

Lost activities	Totally lost?	How might I carry out this activity in my present condition?

Lost characteristics	Totally lost?	Are there positive or useful aspects with the present characteristic?

Exercise 30
Things That Are Authentically Me

Directions: Do this exercise over an extended period of time. Try completing items in the morning, in the afternoon, and in the evening. Examine the exercise when you're feeling relatively full of energy and when you're tired. Fill it in several times and compare your copies. Do your evaluations still feel authentically real to you? Discuss the things that are authentically you with others—your partner, your friends, your counselor. Ultimately, however, write down only what *you* feel is true.

List items for each category. Say why each relationship/activity is important to you.

Activities	Why is this activity important to me?

Relationships With partner	Why is this relationship important to me?
With children (identify)	
With family members (identify)	
With friends	

Exercise 30
Things That Are Authentically Me *continued*

Relationships With co-workers	Why is this relationship important to me?
Work activities	**Why is this activity important to me?**
Personality characteristics	**Why is this personality characteristic important to me?**

Beliefs	Why is this belief important to me?

listener. Being in nature, like experiencing music, can forge a direct creative connection to your spirit, bypassing words altogether.

Stories of heroic captivity. You've probably at some point felt imprisoned by your illness. It's as though someone has locked you in jail, from which you can only peer out through the bars at normal people going about their free lives. If you're a reader, you can learn to use this "imprisonment" by reading the accounts of famous prisoners like Nelson Mandela or Martin Luther King. These men used their time in captivity to grow politically, socially, and spiritually. These are grand stories about issue reframing. These men did not see themselves solely as convicts, but used their time to refine their thinking and expand their understanding.

Folk tales and legends. Many stories exist of people who were forced to live in great adversity but came through to lead meaningful lives. Folk tales, legends, and children's stories can remind you of important qualities that sustain people in times of difficulty or trouble. Often the heroes in these tales suffer difficulty and pain, neglect or hostility, but persist in their quest until they succeed, sometimes with the help of apparently insignificant others whom they were once able to help. These stories can help you increase your ability to reframe issues. You need to see yourself in these roles because you, too, are undergoing an arduous quest. You're seeking out a new self that will give your life meaning and fullness. This new person is going to be someone who is both authentically you and whom you can honor and admire.

Meaning development. As you reframe your experience, as you maintain your insight, as you identify the essential aspects of your new self, as you engage in creative activity, and as you grapple with the big existential questions, you develop meaning. It is this meaning that makes it possible for you to lead a full, rounded life despite your illness. I will discuss this further in "Coping and Comfort."

Humor. Finally, when you're in the pit of despair, the tunnel of desperation, the dark night of the soul, it's hard to see how humor can play a role. But humor, even black humor about how horrible your situation is, can move your work forward. Laughing loosens up your physical and emotional muscles. This is never a matter of making cruel fun of yourself, but rather a matter of seeing the absurdities of life. It makes a great difference if you've got friends or a clinician who can laugh with you. Never miss an opportunity to laugh—laughing is a life-saver.

Taking Control in Your Wider World

Being a burden. In phases one and two you and others in your life mostly believed, even if you did so secretly, that you were going to get better. Of course, how long you'd been sick made you worry about how much trouble you were causing them and whether they'd stick with you despite the difficulties. Indeed, the difficulties of your being ill may have caused significant people from your former life to leave. They probably couldn't deal with the fact that you didn't return to "normal" fast enough. So you had good reason to worry.

In phase three, you've finally recognized that your situation isn't ever going to change, so you may be more worried than ever about being a "burden." It's important for you to know that you are not a burden. You're simply a person with certain needs and requirements, just like everybody else, healthy or sick. You need to talk candidly with the people close to you in order to work out ways to live together. You must answer your needs in ways that don't deplete the significant people in your life.

As early as phase one, but particularly in phase two, you began talking with the people in your life about roles and responsibilities. You began trying to rearrange these to fit with your new realities. Sometimes this meant that everyone had to give up certain past activities. And as I noted, probably you had significant people who just couldn't adjust to the new situation, despite wedding vows or other solemn promises. By phase three you know that you must surround yourself with people who can relate to you as you are. They must be willing to make the effort to work in the world you have to inhabit. Remember, authentic feelings and sincere involvement are part of the bedrock on which you're constructing your new life. You don't want to rely on faulty foundations.

Your situation arouses fear and depression in others. As the important people in your life come to the same recognition you have—that your condition is permanent—their reactions can be similar to yours. They can become afraid, even terrified, or depressed. They feel inadequate to the task and don't know whether they can live with the situation. Anyone can pitch in for an emergency, but forever is another matter. People may be apprehensive about living in the situation with you; they're sometimes scared that something similar might happen to them. Depending on your illness, those close to you most likely fear that they may lose you to death at any moment. Rather than trying to work through this emotional nightmare, they may choose to flee it. Some friends will withdraw from you now. Even your partner may leave. Such separations can be temporary, but they can also be total, permanent losses.

Others experience a dark night of the soul. Like you, the people important to you confront many of the same existential questions you do. Why has this awful thing happened? What's the point of a life where such bad things happen to good people? What kind of a universe permits such things? Like you, they may not have thought deeply about these things before. Whatever religious or philosophical training they received as children may never have been put to the test before. They don't know what to think or how to feel. All they know is that they're adrift and in despair, just like you are.

Working together with your social network. Those close to you will have to work out their issues of meaning individually, just as you do, although they can certainly benefit by using the same techniques. What you can and must do with each other is to establish methods of working out together the ever-changing issues in your lives. One set of arrangements regarding roles and responsibilities, for example, may be needed early in your illness. If you've got small children and you're bedridden, you've got to make new arrangements for the proper care of the children. But perhaps as time goes on, your circumstances change. Children grow up and become more responsible. Your symptoms may plateau in a way that permits you to be up and about more of the day. You and your significant others have to create ways to talk with each other so that you all can readjust to changing conditions. It can be very useful to revisit Exercise 21, "Household Values Clarification and Norm Development," periodically, as your household situation evolves. If you feel that the attitudes of people in your family or your partner are changing, you may want to complete Exercise 9 and 10 again.

Talking meaningfully with each other obviously applies to partners and spouses. But it's equally important between parents and children. Parents with chronically ill children need to recognize that as sick children mature, and if the illness permits, they need to participate as equals, and finally as chiefs, in the management of their illness.

Friends, too, need to recognize that your illness situation is dynamic. It may not be possible for you to socialize publicly at all during some periods. You may have to keep the friendship alive with phone calls or e-mail. But at other times, you may be well enough to thoroughly enjoy a dinner out or a movie together. The key is understanding that chronic illnesses are dynamic and that you and your significant others have to have methods of retooling your interactions as the situation changes.

Change of supporters. Without question, most chronically ill people develop a new set of supporters during their illness. It's so difficult for people to understand and adapt to many chronic illnesses that you doubtless find it easier to place your faith and trust in people like yourself. Other sufferers of chronic illness know what's going on without your having to explain everything. And they're sympathetic, not critical. Many phase three individuals have built up a significant new network of friends who have known them only since they became sick.

You and political action. Many phase three individuals also become politicized by their illness. They're angry at society's ignorance or outright stigmatization. They're distressed that some doctors refuse to consider their illness as legitimate. They're upset at the lack of research into their condition. You may feel the same way and may be more than ready to campaign for your illness support group. Even people who are housebound can address envelopes or send computer messages. Working with a community of engaged individuals, fighting for something you really care about, can inject a whole new sense of purpose into your life.

Reintegration of old supporters. As you gain the self-esteem and greater confidence that characterizes phase three, you may well attempt to reintegrate old friends or family members back into your life. People leave at different times during your illness. In your crisis period some back away because they're too frightened or confused to help. They may have put distance between themselves and you because they were afraid of doing something wrong. Or maybe they were just cowardly.

As you stabilized in phase two, others have left. Some can't take the fact that you continue to be ill. Others leave because they can't stand the change in their own lives. Still others may have different reasons. You have probably been sad, hurt, and angry that these people weren't there when you needed them.

In phase three, however, you understand that it can be very difficult to face problems like yours. These lost family or friends may even have matured since their initial defection but may be awkward about being the one to make the first move. So now you may feel like trying to reestablish contact with them once more.

Some of these old supporters will respond wholeheartedly. They may have learned more than they knew in the past. And they can see that you're willing and able to be friends, even if it's not exactly in the same way as it was in the past. But others won't. If you make an effort to reconnect with people, and they don't want to make the return effort, you should just let the relationship go. It's self-destructive for you to keep trying to have a relationship with people who don't respond to you.

Work issues. If you're still working, the greater self-confidence that you achieve in phase three makes it possible for you to address many of your workplace issues on your own. You're far more likely to speak directly with your employer about your rights under the Americans with Disabilities Act. You're also apt to be more direct about negotiating job arrangements that you can sustain.

You should be prepared for the possibility that you may have to renegotiate arrangements periodically. You can't always have just one discussion, arrive at more satisfactory conditions, and then have these arrangements last forever. Your health status may change, your workplace supervisors may change, the organization itself may go through changes. Any number of things may make it necessary for you to renegotiate your job arrangements several times.

In phase one you probably used a lot of time in sick leave, either because you were ill in bed or because you were seeing doctors. In phase two you may have gone on temporary disability. You may have sought help from your counselor to have workplace interventions that made your job situation more manageable. By phase three you've got a much better concept of what you are physically and cognitively capable of doing over a long period of time. If you can still work, you may decide that it is better for your health to work part-time.

By phase three you may have decided that even part-time work is too exhausting. You need to apply for permanent disability if you have not done so already. You also need to address the issue of finances if you haven't already done so. It's almost always better for you to apply for disability with the help of an experienced counselor rather than attempt to do so on your own. It is probably also wise for you to talk with a professional about your financial situation. You're probably not as thoroughly knowledgeable about tax or savings issues, for example, as people who make it their life's work.

Coping and Comfort

Meeting suffering with respect. You've learned to *allow* your suffering, and you've also begun to regard your suffering with *compassion*. In phase three it's important to regard your suffering with *respect*. Suffering was once the thing you most hated and rejected. But through your unavoidable exposure to it, you've gained unexpected insights and depth. Suffering was nothing you sought or wanted, but now you see that this hated thing has contributed something. By the sheer fact of your endurance, you've grown into a person who is more authentically you than you ever were in the past. You respect yourself for your endurance, for the time you have spent in the dark tunnel.

Heroic captivity. I want to return to the notion of heroic captivity, because that is what your suffering has been. The painful prison to which your illness has committed you becomes a kind of holy ground because it is here that you've constructed a new self, searching and finding a greater, more profound understanding of life. Your suffering and your captivity have become the location of your transformation.

Your personal development of meaning. It may seem odd to say that enduring the dark night and searching for meaning provides comfort and a method of coping. But it does, because the understandings of being and purpose that you find allow you to live beyond your illness. Your private, utterly authentic sense of meaning dissolves the prison walls. You may have to spend a great deal of time dealing with your illness, but it doesn't define you. Your life becomes fuller than that.

In fact, meaning development isn't a task you carry out once and then it's over. For the rest of your life, you'll continue to add to and revise and revisit your beliefs as your experience with life gives you new insights and as you strive to live authentically day to day.

Authenticity drives the search. As you think about the big questions of life and its purpose, you should measure every idea and every belief you encounter against your deepest, most authentic feelings. Does this idea, this belief, ring absolutely true when struck against your feelings? You may have great fondness for traditional beliefs that you've grown up with, and you may resonate to traditional services or ceremonies that you've attended since childhood. You may continue to enjoy participating in such ceremonies, but if the beliefs underneath don't strike true with your deepest feelings, then you want to keep them as part of your culture but not part of your personal meaning. Meaning must be absolutely true for you.

Investigating other traditions. Most people don't know much about what other cultures and traditions have to say about the deep issues of life. Perhaps you feel that you don't even know much about your own culture or religion. As you explore the issues of being and purpose, of suffering and tragedy, you'll gain a lot of insight by learning how cultures other than your own regard these issues. Try talking with people of other spiritual and philosophical traditions. Try visiting spiritual centers—churches, synagogues, mosques, prayer groups, temples— other than those you grew up with. Read about many different spiritual and philosophical approaches to the most important issues of life, meaning, and suffering. You may not agree with what you read, but even so, it gives you a new angle of vision.

Perhaps you're familiar with Christian or Jewish traditions. You might then benefit from reading how Buddhists conceive of the purpose of suffering or how early Greek philosophers regarded the purpose of life. Many contemporary philosophers propose that people assert meaningfulness in their lives by behaving in ways that make life better for themselves and those around them. Folktales from all cultures and all times comment importantly on what it means to be human and why and how people should live.

Nonverbal experiences may help you build a sense of meaning. Perhaps words and discussions have often caused you pain or misunderstanding. If that's the case, nonverbal approaches may come to you as more pure expressions of meaning. Music can reach directly into your visceral perception of the universe and transform it for you in much the same way that mystics are said to be transformed by momentary perceptions of Oneness or God. The diminishing or disappointing associations of words and arguments don't interfere. Or perhaps contemplation of the natural world offers you a vision of such transcendent majesty and beauty that it suffuses you with respect for your existence as part of it.

Internalized, authentic cosmology. Whatever meaning you discover, the test is its internal, authentic truth for you personally. You may continue to participate with great pleasure and satisfaction in your traditional religious practices—you may find your authentic meaning located right there. Or you may have no formal religious framework at all. But inside yourself is a sense of meaning that is absolutely, unquestionably authentic to you. This vision subtly changes as your life proceeds, for the contemplation of meaning never ceases.

Standing with yourself. By the end of phase three, you are willing to stand with yourself. You don't hide who you are or apologize for your existence. You value yourself as a worthwhile human being—indeed, as a heroic soul—who has many things to contribute to the world. Your new self is built on a thoughtful foundation of meaning and draws from all the authentic aspects of your old self which you choose to incorporate.

Integrating the Whole

In phase three your goal is to maintain insight, develop meaning, and construct a new self. Your strategy for doing this is to seek meaning in the tunnel. Physically, illness permitting, you assume management of your physical care. Although your condition is dynamic and may shift and change, you're now able to act as your own care coordinator, health-care advocate, and activities monitor. Psychologically, you cope with your grief and loss. You define your pre-crisis self, and then apply all your developing skills of insight, issue reframing, and creative activity to construct a new self. You analyze what exactly you've lost and what you haven't. Your creative activity helps you begin to develop meaning, which in turn becomes the container for preserving and maintaining your insight. In building your new self and developing meaning, authenticity is the key and the bedrock. You don't pretend any longer. You commit to exploring the painful existential questions that arise when you finally acknowledge that your condition is permanent. Although the process may seem hopeless at the start, you commit to the search for meaning. Using antithetical experimentation and creative activities, you explore who you are now and how that person relates to the person you used to be. In your social world, you assert that you're not a burden, but simply a person with particular needs. You and your significant others find ongoing methods to adapt to the changing conditions of your life together. You rely on supporters who share your experience and value you, although you may also try to reincorporate old friends or family members. You may take up political action related to your illness. You meet your suffering with respect, and you stand with yourself, without apology.

But your most important activity in phase three is your search for meaning that is profoundly true for you personally.

You're now entering phase four, the integration phase, which I'll discuss in the next chapter. This doesn't mean that you've arrived at the perfect life, without any difficulties or setbacks. Nor does it mean that you'll stay there forever. New crises in different areas of your life may force you to revisit earlier phases. But you've come to understand the phases very well and learned how to use them to more forward. You've also integrated a new self and reconstructed your various roles and relationships. In phase four you'll learn how to seek a new "personal best." You'll consciously commit to the daily acts of bravery necessary to your present life. You'll keep up your personal narrative and continue your creative activity. And you'll continue and broaden your search for meaning. All these things will help you construct a rewarding and sustaining life.

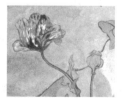

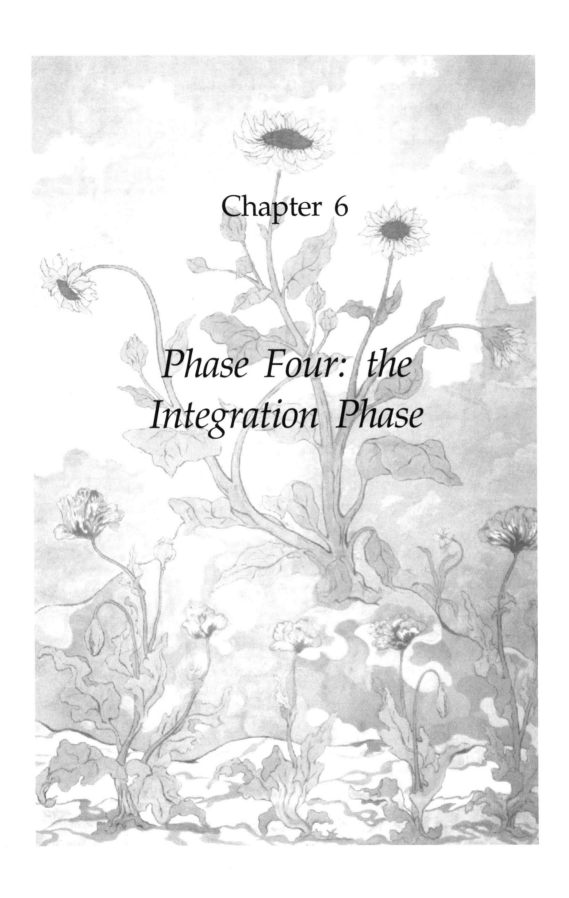

Chapter 6

Phase Four: the Integration Phase

In phase four you integrate your illness into a whole and meaningful life. You no longer live as an illness personified but as an individual with a variety of interests and engagements. This is true even if you're limited physically. Your illness is just one aspect of your being.

This does not mean that you arrive at a perfect life without pain, suffering, frustration, or stigmatization. But it does mean that you've learned how to live graciously in the effort, despite the rigors of life and your particular illness. If the effort you have to make is great, then you value yourself even more for your sheer persistence.

You probably won't live in phase four constantly. Most people experience it only transiently, although sometimes for extended periods. Pain, exhaustion, or the multiplying problems of your illness can wear you down, making you reexperience some of the confusions and distress of earlier phases. Unrelenting pain can dissolve all aspects of humanity if it isn't treated appropriately. Pain management can be a problem for some chronically ill people because they react badly to so many medications. It is important to work with your medical team if you have serious, persistent pain.

Also, despite your awareness of media stigmatization or iatrogenic traumatization, persistent exposure to either one can be deeply distressing. They can cause you to question the understandings that you thought you had reached at the end of phase three.

Finally, life can bring other tragedies or illnesses that knock you back into crisis. Living with chronic illness is a dynamic process, not a static one, even when you've successfully moved through the phase process.

Nonetheless, you can experience true transcendence of your illness in phase four. You're able to construct a three-dimensional life, which includes relationships and social interactions as well as experiences of personal fulfillment. You can do this despite consciousness of your suffering and the chronic, ambiguous nature of your condition.

You can tell that you have entered phase four when you observe the following things to be true about yourself.

Integration

You understand the phases. If you're in phase four, you grasp the concept that recovery, stabilization, and relapse are all parts of the normal cycle of chronic illness. You recognize that integrating your illness into a complete life is an ongoing process. You know that you've learned techniques that you can use to contain future crises, achieve stabilization, and process through resolution to integration again. You also know when and how to seek professional help.

You integrate your pre- and post-crisis selves. In phase four you've constructed a new self. You've redefined yourself, requiring authenticity for every aspect of your new self. In the process, you've incorporated characteristics of your pre-crisis self that you value. You've discarded the harmful scripts that the culture has thrust upon you. You've rewritten your illness story.

You reconstruct your cultural roles and relationships. Because you've made a new self, you've got a very different relationship to your community and your culture. It's a self that includes some characteristics from what you were before your illness. You've integrated some of the "you" from before your illness into the self you are now. In your relations with others, you include, without apology, the reality of your chronic disabilities. The significant others with whom you maintain relationships respond appropriately or ask how to behave if they don't know what is appropriate. Your social roles are varied, and the expenditure of effort they require fits within your activity boundaries.

You now seek broader meaning. In phase four you extend your continuous exploration of meaning outward—more "horizontally," so to speak—to include the world at large. Your interest isn't just "vertical." It doesn't focus solely on your own personal relationship to the universe.

You seek a fuller life. Phase four involves constantly seeking to lead as full a life as possible. You refuse to be defined by your illness. As you expand your life, you recognize the importance of balancing the four broad areas of activity, and you do so without exhausting yourself.

You understand the likelihood of future crises. In phase four you know that your experiences of integration and even transcendence will eventually come under assault from other life crises or different illnesses. But you also know that you have learned powerful and successful techniques for integrating these future crises. Given the longer lives that most Americans can expect to live, you know that you're likely to become sick with other illnesses. You're as vulnerable as others to accidents or the loss of loved ones. You're as frightened of these prospects as everyone is and perhaps with better reason, given your experiences. However, you also know how to live daily in the present and how to work with your fears and griefs. On good days, you do just that. On bad days, you hang onto your new faith that you know how to work toward better days.

Strategy: Achieving a Full and Rewarding Life

Goal. The goal of phase four is to integrate your suffering into a meaningful, sustaining, and rewarding life. Once again you accomplish this through tactics and skills addressed to your physical self, your psychological self, and yourself in relation to others.

Living wisely in the now. Physically, you constantly attune your life to the changing demands of your body, which you maintain with regular medical and activity reviews.

Growing creatively and spiritually. Psychologically, you continue and deepen the work you began in phase three. In particular, you continue to engage in creative activity and meaning development.

Expanding your social horizons. Socially, you refine your maintenance reviews with your family, partner, or friends so that you can adjust to changes in your circumstances. You also expand your social life and continue to participate in social action. If you still have a work life, phase four is often the time when you change your occupation completely in order to make it more congruent with the requirements of your new, authentic self. Even if you stopped formal employment some time ago, you may find that you want to volunteer such service as you can to a cause you think is important.

Tactics and Skills

Living Wisely in the Now

Attuning yourself to your illness cycles. By phase four you've acquired a great deal of experience with your illness. You've probably been through two or more cycles of plateau followed by relapse and then slow improvement. You've learned to pay attention to your symptoms. If they worsen significantly or take a completely new form, you see your doctor immediately. At the same time you begin cutting back on all areas of activity until the physical crisis is contained. As you improve and stabilize, you know how to add activities back into your life in a way that doesn't strain you physically.

Maintaining medical reviews. You maintain a regular schedule of medical reviews, making sure to get whatever tests are necessary to continue to receive disability, if you're receiving disability. You pay attention to your reactions to medications and other medical protocols and draw your doctor's attention to areas where you believe there is difficulty. You keep yourself informed about new developments in the treatment of your illness so that you can bring these up with your medical team. Your primary doctor is usually a generalist who cannot stay abreast of all medical research. It is incumbent upon you to keep track of new findings and treatments that may help alleviate or improve your condition.

Maintaining activity reviews. You regularly review your activities and activity levels. In part you do this so that your activities fit the changing circumstances of your life. But you also do it so that you can think about whether you're allocating your energy to activities that are meaningful and rewarding for you. Many people don't pay attention to how they spend their time. They just do what they've always done, sometimes adding a new sport or recreational activity. But you've learned that the quality of your life is affected by everything that you do. You want all your activities to contribute to the highest quality of life you can achieve.

Growing Creatively and Spiritually

Maintaining your personal narrative. Your own story is one of your strongest methods for staying conscious of what you're doing in your life and how you feel about it. If you have been writing this story as a narrative, you may change the format when you enter phase four. You may decide to keep a journal or diary rather than continuing to recast a narrative of your entire life. You're sufficiently familiar with the important episodes in your past so that you can see how they fit into current situations quite readily. If you've been making audiotapes of your story, you may want to turn this into a sort of spoken diary. Perhaps you prefer to paint or draw or sculpt representations of your evolving understanding of your life. How you maintain your personal narrative is limited only by your imagination.

Maintaining your new self and your new "personal best." In phase three you constructed a new self based on what you could be, what was authentic, and characteristics from your pre-crisis self that you wanted to keep. Living in phase four means that you maintain and improve this new self. You set goals, a new "personal best," which you actively seek to achieve as much of the time as possible. You don't settle for a second-rate life. You don't regard yourself as some sort of damaged, lesser person who can't expect much of yourself. Instead, you work to be the best person you can be.

Exercising free will. You choose to do everything that you take on. It is your free will that drives you to carry out your daily acts of bravery. You do this despite the fact that your many small (or large) courageous acts receive no notice, and you receive no recognition or honor for them. This is very hard work. It requires daily attention and self-discipline. But by persisting in the effort, you constantly build self-respect, and the self-respect in turn helps you persist in the effort. You set in motion a positive cycle in which disciplined persistence increases your self-respect, and your self-respect enables you to continue persisting.

Continuing creativity. The creative impulse in everyone ebbs and flows. Sometimes you'll experience times of great imaginative richness, but at other times the impulse will slacken and you'll have little drive to create. It's very rare, however, for people to stop altogether once they've begun seeking and growing and creating. With your eyes opened and your search begun, you'll almost surely continue to create periodically for the rest of your life.

Continuing meaning development. The same is true for meaning development. Once you've begun thinking about the most essential questions of being and purpose, it's highly unlikely that you'll ever stop. Meaning development and refinement enriches your ever-changing present. In the best moments of phase four, your sense of meaning spreads out to encompass all aspects of your everyday life as well as your relationship to the universe. You find value and even honor in the simple tasks of daily living. Relationships become important simply for being relationships—for being a space where love, kindness, and service occur.

You no longer look solely at what the universe is in relation to you. You pay attention to what it must be in relation to everyone in the world. You think about how you contribute to the world around you. You pay attention to what you can do to make life better and more meaningful for others. In phase four, you may volunteer in some activity that seeks to improve the lives of others.

You ground your sense of meaning—you make it real and actual—by observing it operate in all four areas of activity in your life. You come to see meaning in the small tasks of your ADLs. Meaning casts a new light on your work activities. Meaning deepens and enriches your many different social relations. And of course, the philosophical and spiritual growth that creates this meaning illuminates your activities of personal fulfillment.

Expanding Your Social Horizons

Evaluating and revising your family/partner/friend maintenance reviews. In phase three, you and the other significant people in your life worked out ways to review your living arrangements with each other. Because life is constantly changing, these reviews need to be flexible and capable of adjustment. Periodically you'll need to talk with those closest to you about whether the systems you've got in place are functioning the way they should.

Continuing social action. You'll probably continue to pursue social action in relation to your illness or issues related to it. Such activity not only improves the experience of others who suffer and helps to change negative cultural perceptions, but it's also very invigorating for you, even if you're severely disabled. It also usually involves you with others who share and understand your experiences.

Recruiting and maintaining "integrated" supporters. In phase three you began to develop a strong network of new supporters. These people acknowledge and accept the real life that you live now. They understand your limits but don't consider the fact that you have limitations to be an impediment to intimacy and engagement. You may also have begun reaching out to former friends and family members from whom you were distanced when you first became ill. If these people have learned to understand your situation or are willing to learn, then you'll probably reintegrate them into your life. Long-term relationships have a value all their own, which most people want to preserve if they can.

Workplace or vocational changes. You try to live as authentically as you can. You try to make your life as meaningful as possible. As a consequence, you're no longer satisfied just to earn wages if you still work. You want to work at something that you believe has value and importance. Many people change their careers at the end of phase three or during phase four.

Perhaps you've been unable to work at all or have only worked occasionally. In phase four you may decide that you want to participate more actively in society by volunteering your services to some cause that you support. Even if you must spend most of your time in bed, you may be able to make phone calls or stuff envelopes or perform other desperately needed services for a good cause. Contributing to the welfare of society can raise your spirits fantastically.

Coping and Comfort

Integration of suffering. In phase four you integrate your suffering into your life. It's there, so you intentionally and consciously include it as part of your life. You have, in the phase process, gone through a progression. In phase one you allowed that your suffering existed. You acknowledged that it was there. Phase two involved permitting yourself to feel compassion for your suffering. You came to respect your suffering in phase three because you learned important things from it, because it caused you to grow, but most of all because you endured it. Now, in phase four, you integrate your suffering as an aspect, but only one aspect, of your life.

Daily acts of bravery. Achieving phase four doesn't relieve you of pain, suffering, or difficulty. You've got to commit yourself to acting bravely every day. Every day you'll probably face some assault on your courage and good intentions. Besides what your body does to you, you'll continue to face instances of stigmatization. You'll have to continue to assert your worthiness in the face of indifference, dismissal, and sometimes outright malice. Even your friends can be hurtful, though they do it in ignorance. Moreover, you're constantly having to assert to yourself that you're not taxing your partner or your family. You're going to stumble in the process of dealing with all of this. But you're also going to persist. Odd as it may seem, acting bravely, even if you don't necessarily feel brave, will give you comfort and raise your self-esteem.

Social and creative action. Both your social action and your creative activities help you cope with the day-to-day difficulties of living with chronic illness. They can also provide great comfort. Your social action puts you in contact with like-minded people and helps improve the lives of others. Your creative activities continuously demonstrate to you that even if you must live in a very unsatisfactory physical situation, you can add richness and substance to your life. The time you spend engaged in creation also takes you out of yourself into a kind of meditative state that heals and sustains your spirit as you develop your skill in making new things.

Increased awareness of meaning at all levels. Your ongoing attention to issues of meaning make you look at all aspects of your life and the lives of those around you differently from the way you did before you became ill. More and more, you see that everything about your life has meaning. The most insignificant aspect or action—how you make your bed, how you sit or stand when you're talking with someone—can have meaning. And when you feel that it does, you enrich your life and the lives of those around you. In phase four you know that meaning affects how you do everything, how you treat everyone, and how you think about yourself. Meaning founded on your authentic inner sense of truth surrounds and suffuses your waking hours. You come to meaning as a way of coping, and meaning in your life allows you to cope more satisfactorily with difficulties in the future. As you build a whole life, your personal philosophical and spiritual perceptions enrich it.

Living with paradox. When you reach phase four you're able to live with the paradox of a full life lived with compromised health. You've got an illness that may be very debilitating and limiting, but you're able to accept this fact and still lead a full and three-dimensional life. You're strengthened by faith in yourself because you've proven to yourself that you can endure *and* find a better place. Yours is not some mindless faith. You've had many rough times, and you're aware you'll have them in the future. But you also know that you can survive and move on because you've done it before. This isn't a clenched-teeth approach to life. Although you deal with pain and suffering when they occur, the rest of the time you focus on meaningful activities that enrich your existence. You can lead a full life despite the chronicity and ambiguity of your illness.

Living in the mystery. However it is that you've arrived there, you've learned to live in the mystery of a universe where very bad things can happen to good people—or even just ordinary people. But it's also a place where you see people rising magnificently to the occasion out of the most stressful of difficulties. With no prospect of gain or reward, apparently unremarkable people do brave, selfless, and loving things. Awareness that reasons in the universe are largely unknowable doesn't disable you with depression or anger because you've found meaningful ways to live in the world. This is not to say that you never doubt or question, that you never throw up your hands. You're constantly in the process of reacting to life and of reflecting on and modifying your conception of meaning.

A Place of Integration

When you're in phase four—and it's rare to remain there constantly—your goal is to integrate your illness into a whole and meaningful life. You're not without pain and symptoms, but you've learned how to live graciously in the effort. Physically, you live wisely in the now. You're attuned to your illness cycle so you know when significant changes occur. You maintain your medical reviews and keep abreast of developments in your illness. You also maintain activity reviews to make sure that your activities fit the changes in your life. Psychologically, you continue to grow creatively and spiritually. You keep on writing your personal narrative, in part as a way to remain conscious about what you're thinking and what you're doing. You've integrated your pre- and post-crisis selves and maintain your new self. You establish a new "personal best." You regard your daily acts of bravery as matters of free will, and you feel growing self-respect for your ability to endure. You continue to engage in creative activity and meaning development. Philosophically and spiritually, you look not only to yourself but to your whole world, from the smallest tasks to universal considerations. You expand your social horizons as much as your condition will permit. You continuously seek to keep in touch with your relationships with family, partner, and friends, and you also recruit new supporters and integrate old ones who wish to reconnect to your life. When possible, you continue to engage in social action. And in your work or vocational life, you strive for authentically meaningful work activities. You've integrated suffering into your life, not because you like it but because you must live with it. You're aware of the bravery you exhibit day by day and this awareness helps increase and sustain your self-esteem. You find that meaning suffuses all life, including yours. You may be living in a paradox, but you can do this, just as you can live in the mystery of a world where bad or difficult things happen to good people. You're constantly in the process of revising your concepts of meaning, but always you keep in mind the knowledge that you are, no matter how limited, a valuable person who is worthy of love.

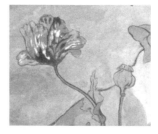

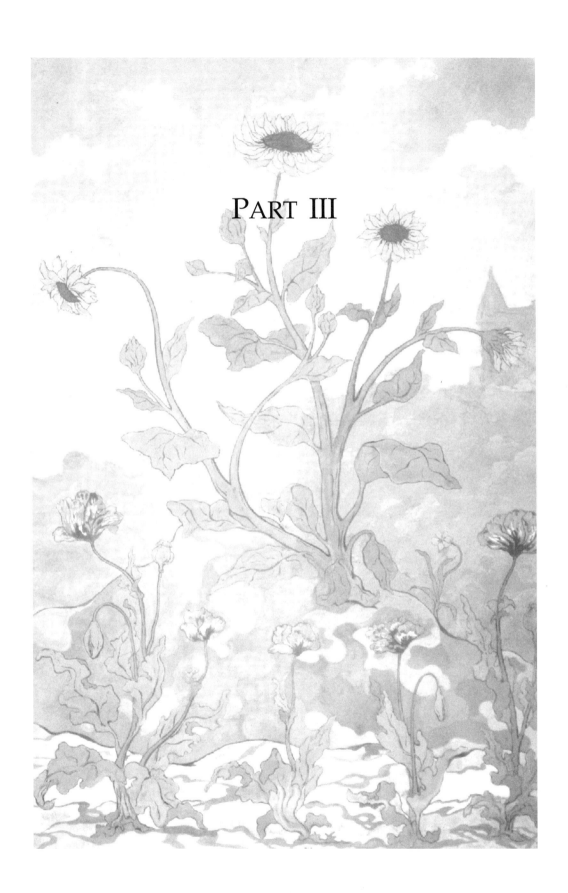

PART III

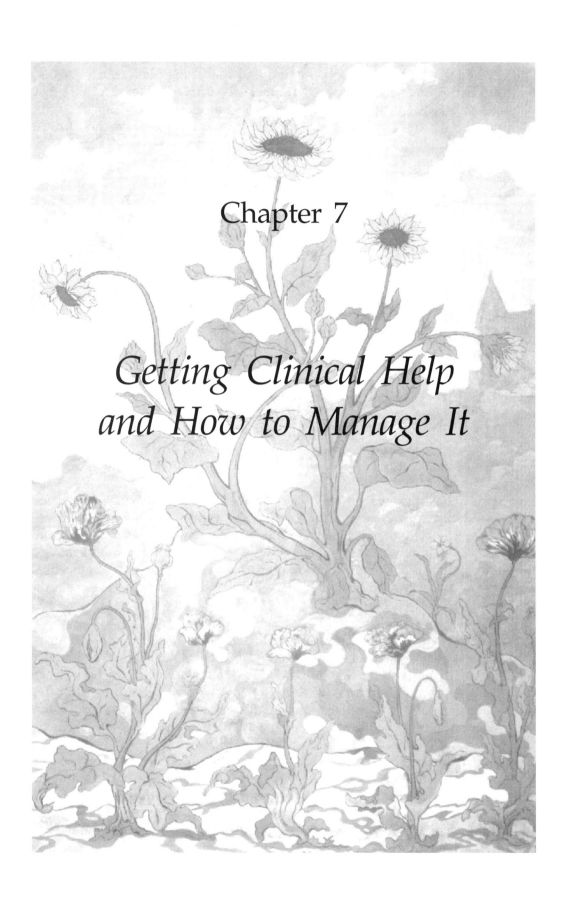

Chapter 7

*Getting Clinical Help
and How to Manage It*

I've covered some material about getting and managing clinical help earlier, but this chapter puts it all together in one place for easy reference. Whether you're the person with the chronic illness, or you're caring for someone with a chronic illness, you're going to have a lot of contact with health-care professionals. So you've got to know how to find them, what to look for, and how to deal with them when you get them.

What to Look For

Qualified Professionals

Qualifications. Your doctors, psychologist, social worker, physical therapist, occupational therapist, or sleep specialist all should be qualified professionals. These people should be licensed and required to have certain levels of training. The American Medical Association, for example, has a directory of all doctors in the country, whether they are members of AMA or not, available on its Web site (www.ama-assn.org). The directory is organized by medical specialty. In addition to the doctors' names, addresses, and phone numbers, the AMA provides information on where the doctors trained, when they graduated, where they did their residencies and in what specialty. Most medical specialties have their own associations and certification programs as well. Sleep studies should be conducted only at certified sleep clinics.

State licensing departments. If you want details of what competencies you should expect of doctors, psychologists, therapists, social workers, massage therapists, acupuncturists, etc., you can contact the department in your state that licenses these professionals. They will tell you what qualifications people in that field are required to demonstrate before they receive a license. They can also give you information on how the state monitors the standards of those already licensed.

Alternative providers. The lack of verified qualifications and standards monitoring are two problems with using alternative health-care providers. Some alternative providers are very good. They listen to their patients closely and spend considerable time with them. People who've been put off by the clinical distance and chill of some conventional medical practices find such personal attention healing in itself. Other patients seek out alternative practitioners when conventional medical care is not bringing about the changes they seek in their physical and psychological condition. But since anyone can set up office as an alternative healer, you're vulnerable to harmful treatment or fraud when you opt for alternative treatment. If you drop conventional care when you take up alternative treatment, you may well be seriously endangering what health you have. Be extremely careful if you pursue alternative treatments.

Professionals You Like and Trust

Liking the professionals. Since most people will actually find their way to qualified professionals, at least when they begin trying to identify and treat their chronic illness, what's really important is locating clinicians whom you like and trust. You know that you like people when they listen to you, are interested in you, pay attention to what you say, treat you with respect, and demonstrate a caring attitude toward you. You can measure liking for your doctor in the same way. It's extremely important for anyone with a chronic illness to like their doctors and other health-care providers. You're going to see them a lot.

Trusting them. Trusting your caregivers is just as important as liking them, but trust is built over time. Trust comes about as you see that your clinicians have been completely candid with you about what they understand of your condition and how they're going to treat it. When one approach doesn't help, trustworthy clinicians acknowledge that it's not helping you and consider other options. If they're confused or unsure, they're able to say so without distancing themselves from you or blaming you. They are able to stay in the process with you. They anticipate that they will meet treatment obstacles and setbacks, and they manage their disappointment if it occurs. If they find they can't grapple with your problem effectively, they refer you to other professionals who may be able to help. If the referring doctor is your primary physician, he or she makes sure to keep abreast of what happens to you with the referral doctor.

Professionals who believe you. Finally, make sure to see professionals who believe you and take your opinion seriously. In addition to dealing with your illness, you don't want to have to struggle with doctors or other professionals who don't believe what you're saying. Some clinicians go by the book. They've read what symptoms people with your condition ought to have and so they pay attention to this "knowledge" rather than what you actually report. They don't consider that the books may have faulty or incomplete information, and that you're telling them what is really happening to you as an individual with this illness.

Some clinicians don't believe reported symptoms when they can't see measurable proof that the symptoms have occurred or are occurring. You have to have a fever right then in the office or a rash or be unable to lift your leg several times or be unable to achieve balance on one foot. You can't afford to endure this kind of narrow viewpoint based on an acute model of illness. You need to find clinicians who believe what you tell them.

If you're a caregiver. These characteristics of desirable professionals are equally important if you're not the sick person yourself, but you're caring for the person who's sick. Your care recipient must like and trust the professionals dealing with his or her case. This is obvious with adults, but it's true for children as well. Your sick child should like and feel comfortable with his or her health-care professionals. And whether your care recipient is an adult or a child, you should also feel comfortable with the clinicians. If you don't like or trust a clinician treating the person you're caring for, the chances are great that the person you're caring for doesn't like or trust that clinician either, but is going along with the situation because it seems to be necessary.

Talk with your care recipient about all the professionals you see so that you know that the person you're caring for is comfortable. You also want to observe that the clinicians listen to this person attentively and believe what he or she reports.

How to Find Good Professionals

Use Your Friendship Network

General opinions. If you've been living in your community for some time, try talking to all your friends and asking them to ask their friends about doctors in your community. You can learn a lot from their experiences. You may decide to discount things that one person or another says, and you may have your own assessment of a friend that makes you question how they've evaluated a particular doctor. But you'll definitely get a sense of which doctors listen to their patients and which ones believe their patients. You'll have a good idea of why people like one doctor and don't particularly care for another. You also want to ask them about how the staff in the doctor's office treated them. This will give you a good indication of how the staff will treat you over time, including how they will convey your messages to the doctor.

Specific instances. By asking, you can also learn about specific instances of good treatment or bad treatment. It is extremely hard to get information about whether doctors have been sued for malpractice and the outcomes of those suits. It's equally hard to learn whether doctors have had hospital privileges suspended or have suffered from other problems which affect their ability to practice. Since this is the case, you have to pay attention to specific stories that your friendship network can provide.

When you're new in town. If you're moving to a new location, ask your doctor in your present location to provide the names of doctors and other professionals in the community you're moving to. Your old doctor can at least provide the names of qualified people and may even know personally about specific professionals in your new location. In your new location, ask people at your new workplace to describe their doctors. If you've got any personal friends who live in the area, ask them as well.

Use Your Illness Support Group

If you've already been diagnosed, your illness support group can be a great help in finding professionals who understand your condition and are reported to treat patients with this condition well. If you have a local chapter, you can talk personally with individuals in the group about the various medical personnel in the area. But even if you haven't got a local chapter, usually the national organization can provide the names of doctors who work in your disease area.

A disease support group is invaluable if you've just moved to a new location and know very few people. The national organization may be able to provide names, and if there is a local chapter, you've immediately made some new acquaintances who have all sorts of information about local practitioners.

Warning about Personal Evaluations

Whether they come from friends, people in your workplace, or individuals in your support group, opinions about medical practitioners will be colored by your informant's character and things in that person's experience. In part, of course, that's what you want, since their personal opinion tells you something about how individual professionals relate to their patients and clients. But you should remember that these descriptions don't give you a complete or objective evaluation of the professional. In addition, one person may dislike a doctor whom other people find very competent, considerate, and attentive

Seeking Help from a Medical Social Worker

If you want more objective information, you may find it helpful to contact a medical social worker to discuss your disease and how to go about obtaining the best medical help for it in your location. Although social workers are individuals with personal preferences like the rest of us, they will approach the evaluation of local practitioners more objectively than your friends will. At the same time they're usually aware of which practitioners are interested in your problem, which ones are attentive and believing, and which ones patients have found most helpful.

Social workers also see the big picture of your illness. They may recommend that you contact certain professionals in areas that you hadn't even considered to help with problems related to your illness. If you're new to a location, it can be particularly helpful to consult with a medical social worker about finding appropriate health-care professionals. You can contact the National Association of Social Workers or your local state association in order to get names.

Dealing with HMOs

Primary physician. If you belong to an HMO, you may have a very limited range of doctor choice. Ordinarily you must go through your gatekeeper primary physician to reach other specialists. This makes choosing your primary physician crucially important. Most HMOs have several primaries available, so you should try to locate the one whose manner and attitude best fits with you. It's less important that your primary be an expert on your condition than that he or she is willing to learn and to refer you to specialists as necessary. Remember to pay attention to the office staff as well. They will be important because they mediate your contact with the doctor.

Nurse practitioner. It's also possible that your primary doctor's office has a nurse practitioner. These professionals can often spend more time with you than the doctors can, which means that you can give the kind of complex description of your symptoms that chronic illness usually requires. Many patients state that nurse practitioners have a warm and friendly manner that makes them seem more accessible than doctors often seem. Many times they are able to make referrals or their recommendations for referral are regularly acted upon by the doctors in the office.

Available services. You'll want to learn from your primary physician and from reading your health-care policy what services are available to you and under what conditions. It is really important for you to read your health-care contract and to understand what services your health maintenance organization will provide, for how long, and under what circumstances. What is the HMO's medications prescription policy? Will the HMO allow you to see a specialist outside the organization? Will it allow you to see a specialist in another city or state? If so, what conditions have to be met and what permissions do you need? What's the HMO's policy on physical and occupational therapy? What's their policy on counseling? Can you see a medical/clinical social worker or a psychologist? What kinds of home medical equipment do they help pay for?

When to change HMOs. If you find that your present health insurance won't permit you access to many of the services you need, you should try to change to a health insurance organization that does. Different HMOs provide different service selections, and you may be able to find one that fits your particular needs better.

Services you pay for. It is a fact, however, that certain services that will help you significantly may be ones that you'll have to pay for on your own. However, many aspects of living with chronic illness can be so greatly improved when you receive these services that it's worth the expense. If the cost is totally beyond your budget, a social worker may be able to help you locate publicly funded services.

Expectations

What Should You Expect from Your Doctors?

Go through this checklist with regard to all your health-care providers.

❏ Your doctors should treat you competently, respectfully, and with caring attention.

❏ Your doctors should take the time to listen to you carefully.

❏ Your doctors should demonstrate that they believe what you report to them.

❏ Your doctors should inform you of their findings and diagnoses in language that you understand, and they should make sure that you understand what they have been telling you by asking you questions. Your answers show whether you understand or not.

❏ Your doctors should answer all your questions.

❏ Your doctors should explain what they are going to do and how most people experience the treatment they're prescribing. They should tell you about any regularly anticipated side effects and inform you about what to do if you have unanticipated reactions.

❏ If your doctors aren't able to figure out what's going on with you, they should say so and refer you to other doctors who may be better able to diagnose and treat you.

❏ Your doctors should perform tests on you prudently to determine your condition or when the results will aid in selecting better treatment for you. They should not carry out tests simply because that's the automatic next step.

❏ Your doctors' offices should schedule appointments in such a fashion that you're not kept waiting an unreasonable amount of time if you arrive on time, and you're not rushed when you're with the doctor.

❏ The personnel in your doctors' offices should be respectful and attentive, and they should answer questions clearly and politely.

Asking for Additional Opinions

You should **always** be able to ask for additional opinions with regard to your medical condition. If your doctor rejects your request outright or attempts to discourage you, that's a red flag for you. You should think about changing doctors.

What Your Doctors Expect from You

You've also got obligations. You should act in a spirit of mutual respect with your doctor, being polite, reasonable, and respectful when you're treated with respect. You must report as clearly and completely as possible, even though you may want to be careful about how you phrase what you say (see "Your Medical Record" below).

If you don't understand what your doctor tells you, you must say so. Then you must listen attentively to their explanations until you do understand.

You must attempt to comply with treatment protocols. If you stop a protocol that's been ordered, you should inform your doctor that you've discontinued it and why.

You should meet all your appointments or inform the office in advance if you're not going to be able to make it. Since you want your doctors' attention for the time you are scheduled, you should make sure to arrive on time.

If Clinicians' Behavior Doesn't Meet Expectations

What do you do if your clinicians' behavior doesn't meet your expectations?

Speak out. Sometimes you may simply need to draw attention to the issue. You may be able to say, for example, "I don't understand what you're telling me. Would you please explain it again?" If the doctor immediately rephrases the explanation and answers your questions until you do understand, then you've got a doctor who is trying to treat you the way you should be treated.

If the doctor repeats information you've given in a way that you think changes its meaning, you should correct the doctor's misimpression. If the doctor indicates that he or she recognizes and accepts the correction, this again is a doctor who is trying to work with you appropriately.

If you cry in the doctor's office and the doctor says that you must be feeling depressed, you should be able to discuss this. It's possible that you are depressed. But perhaps you feel you have reasons to cry that do not arise from depression. You and your doctor should be able to talk about either possibility and arrive at a strategy for dealing with it that you both agree upon.

If you've been treated rudely or insensitively by any office personnel, you should be able to mention this to your doctor. In subsequent visits you should find that the staff behave differently.

In all of the above instances, you've been able to say something that permits the doctor or staff to correct their behavior. If they change and attempt to act the way you've got every right to expect, there is good reason to continue with these professionals.

Not feeling free to speak out. If, however, everything about the doctor, the staff, and the office prevents you from being able to speak out, or if they become angry or hostile when you do speak out, then you should immediately seek a new doctor. You can't work effectively with a doctor who behaves in a distant, cold, authoritarian, or dismissive way. No meaningful communication will take place, and without that the doctor will simply not have a proper picture of what's happening to you.

Don't tolerate disrespectful, demeaning, or hurtful behavior. Some kinds of disrespectful, demeaning, and hurtful behavior won't be corrected no matter what you say, and that's often apparent right from the start. If your doctor is regularly disrespectful of you, demeans you, or hurts you, you must change doctors.

Your Medical Record

It's permanent. What's written in your medical record is permanent. It is extremely hard to correct even honest errors in medical records. On the one hand, this protects you, but there are also pitfalls here, especially if you've got a chronic illness. Chronic illnesses are notoriously difficult to describe and assess, and it's easy for even the best-intentioned doctor to write something down that may be damaging for you later, especially if you eventually seek disability.

Essential in claiming disability. Whether you receive disability or not depends very largely on your medical record. It has been argued that those who investigate applications for disability have an economic incentive to add as few new individuals as possible to the lists of those receiving disability, so they'll tend to be looking for reasons why you should be denied. Unfortunately, many doctors don't know what items on your record will make it very difficult for you to make a successful claim. These doctors may even feel that you truly deserve and need disability, but because they don't know about some of the disqualifying issues, they write damaging information into your permanent record. If you believe that you'll need to apply for disability, you want to discuss the issue first with a qualified counselor who knows the area well or talk about it with a lawyer. It may also help you to go to your local illness association or the association's Web site. Many chronic illness associations post articles relevant to application for disability when you've got that particular condition. You can download this material and share it with your doctor.

Accessing and understanding your medical record. You've got a legal right to your medical record. You can and should ask your doctor for a copy.

Actually, the best way to keep up to date with your medical record is to collect copies of your visit report and any lab work that was done at the time of each visit. This way you don't run into the problem of having to ask the staff to copy a huge file all at once.

Read the record and make sure that you understand what it contains, at least in a broad, general way. Your doctor may be willing to spend the time going over it with you, but you may also want to examine it with another informed third party.

Accuracy of your record. Review your record to see whether it accurately reflects your experience. If you feel that it misrepresents what you think is true, you should be able to discuss this with your doctor. Sometimes doctors will add additional information that reflects your experience, but sometimes the only way you can introduce additional information into your record is by seeing a doctor who makes a different evaluation of your condition. That doctor's record then acts to qualify the findings of the first doctor. It's important to remember here that chronic illnesses are notoriously difficult to diagnose because they usually involve an array of shifting symptoms. Many doctors aren't familiar with some chronic illnesses and may well write down an honest but mistaken diagnosis.

Because your record is permanent and can have a profound effect on your ability to obtain disability, be very aware of the impression you make on your doctor. While you should be candid and complete about reporting your symptoms, you may also want to exercise some judgment about how you describe them. It's also important that you think about your demeanor and behavior in the doctor's office. In many instances the doctor notes down information about a patient's attitude and behavior, and this then becomes part of your permanent medical record. Since the assessment of how you're acting or appearing is simply the doctor's interpretation and not some sort of absolute truth, you need to think about what kind of impression you're creating when you're in the doctor's office.

I know that there seems to be a contradiction between being assertive and authentic with your doctor and exercising caution. Appropriate communication is mostly a matter of *how* you present your information. You need to be concise. You need to be objective. You need to be calm. If you ramble or start to cry or talk angrily about your rotten experiences with doctors, the emotional content of such communication may strongly affect how the doctor "hears" the physical symptoms you describe. It may cause the doctor to regard your emotional symptoms as being far more significant than any reported physical symptoms or perhaps even completely responsible for them. Sometimes emotional symptoms *are* the most important symptoms, and represent the truth of the situation. But whether they accurately reflect your condition or not, the doctor's psychological assessments go into your permanent medical records.

How to See Your Doctor

Go prepared. Prior to seeing your doctor, keep track of all the things you want to report and ask. Many people recommend that you write out a list so that you won't forget anything. If you know your doctor well and trust him or her, this is a good idea. But despite many public recommendations that people make lists, some doctors take offense at them, even though they may not seem to. If you're seeing a doctor for the first time, you may want to memorize your list. On the other hand, taking a written list may be a good way to evaluate the doctor's response.

Take a companion. It's always a good idea to see a doctor with a companion whom you trust, especially if it's a first visit or if you're in pain or distress. It's very hard to keep track of what's happening when you're suffering or scared. Having a friend with you taking notes permits you to check after the visit on everything the doctor said. You can also use your friend to help with your list of concerns. If this person is aware of the particular issues you want to bring up, she or he can remind you if you forget something.

Businesslike behavior. Remember, although it's the doctor's business to help you with your medical problems, it's still a business. She or he is not a friend, even though your relations can and should be friendly. The doctor's time is limited, so you should be succinct and to the point about your symptoms. Assess before your visit just what issues you want to bring up, and as difficult as it may be, you should march through them without getting distracted by other personal concerns, unless those concerns are related to your symptoms and should be reported.

Describing your symptoms. Your doctor wants to know the following about your symptoms: When did this begin? How often has or does each occur? How severe is the symptom? In what way does it bother you? You should consider ahead of time, for example, what kind of pain you feel. Is it a sharp stabbing pain? Is it a dull ache? Does it throb? Is it always located in the same place? Does it always occur at the same time? Try to have a clear understanding and explanation of your symptoms to share with your doctor.

Rehearsing. It's often a good idea to practice what you want to say before going to the doctor. Rehearsing is good prior to all sorts of situations where you may be anxious, scared, or just plain shy. By saying out loud ahead of time what your symptoms are and how and when you feel them, the words become familiar. You hear what you're going to say and so when you repeat it in the doctor's office, it's something you've done before. So, even with a new doctor in a strange office, you're at home with what you've got to say.

Alternative Medical Care

Benefits

Attentive practitioners. Many alternative care providers offer help and services that the conventional medical system may ignore, restrict, or disparage. Some spend far more time with clients, engaging with them sympathetically and personally in a broader, more holistic way. This extra attention can help you improve psychologically and socially, which in turn can help you improve physically.

Diet. Many alternative practices pay close attention to diet. Conventional medical providers will sometimes remind patients that they should eat a healthy diet. They may even refer you to a nutritionist, if you request it. But many alternative practitioners work with you week in and week out to arrive at a diet that makes you feel much better.

Pain. Many alternative practitioners work with clients who have intractable pain. Most conventional medicine attempts to deal with pain through medication, short-term physical therapy, or a course of goal-oriented behavior therapy. But some patients have persistent pain because they can't take pain medications without serious side effects or their pain doesn't respond to conventional medication or therapy. It's a sorry fact that some conventional providers become frustrated and annoyed when they're unable to produce the results they believe their medicine should provide. They tend to want to avoid patients who don't respond. On the other hand, some conventional doctors will recommend alternative treatments when their own have failed. Many patients report that their alternative practices do reduce or even eliminate their pain.

Meditation. Many alternative practices include some form of meditation as part of the treatment. For years conventional medicine ignored the benefits of meditation. Eventually conventional medical research discovered that meditation actually produced measurable physical benefits—slowing heart rate, calming emotions—that, in turn, measurably helped improve patients' physical situation. But meditation has only recently been accepted as a treatment within the western model of medicine. Many doctors do not think to include meditation or counseling as part of their treatment plan.

Exercise and massage. Alternative practices often include gentle or low-impact exercise activities that physically challenged people are able to accomplish without pain. Most conventional medical doctors advocate exercise as a way to improve patient well-being, but sometimes the kinds of exercise they're familiar with are too strenuous or painful for patients at a certain point in their chronic illness. You need to report to your doctor any difficulties with any recommended exercise program and work out satisfactory alternatives that you can manage.

Alternative practices may include massage. Among its many other benefits, massage reintroduces touch into the lives of people who may be sorely deprived of this important curative experience. Conventional medical practice rarely includes "touchy-feely" treatment, but this may be precisely what is necessary to relax the client's body so that its own self-regulating mechanisms can be supported.

Spiritual/philosophical component. Alternative practices usually include a spiritual or philosophical component. Dealing with spiritual or philosophical issues is crucial to achieving an integrated life if you have chronic illness, and conventional medicine rarely steps into this territory. If the alternative practice has a spiritual or philosophical component that is truly authentic for you, then it provides an additional healing component.

Drawbacks

Absence of scientifically proven effectiveness. Very few alternative treatments have undergone the kind of empirical scientific testing that conventional medicine requires. As a consequence, claims of effectiveness are based solely on what is called "anecdotal evidence," or individual patient report. Anecdotal evidence is often very suggestive, but it's not proof. When you engage in alternative medicine, you're usually submitting yourself to formally untested, unproven treatment.

Lack of standards or regulation. As mentioned earlier, alternative care is largely unregulated. While massage therapists, for example, are now licensed in some states, anyone may offer "body work" without being licensed. These people may or may not know what they're doing, but without appropriate training they can quite possibly harm you. The very restricted diets of some alternative practices may be denying you nutrients that you need, or may be creating problems that you didn't have before.

Unregulated herbal remedies and dietary supplements. The herbal preparations and dietary supplements that are part of some alternative practices are not required to meet any food or drug regulations. Because at the present time they are unregulated and usually untested, you cannot count on their having any efficacy or even uniformity. Some do not even contain the ingredients they purport to contain, or not in sufficient quantity to be of any use. Others contain more of certain ingredients than appears to be healthy for people to take. The European countries have carried out rigorous testing on the effects of some herbal medicine, but a great deal needs to be done before we can have complete confidence in these remedies.

"Unwillingness to heal." Beware of any practitioner who says or implies that your inability to recover or improve is a reflection of your "unwillingness to heal." Check any feedback of this sort with your friends and others close to you, including your conventional health-care team. It may be an issue worth investigating, or it may be a method a provider uses to cope with unsuccessful outcomes. This is even more pertinent when practitioners indicate that you're unwilling to heal because you haven't purchased some treatment or treatments that they offer.

Spiritual or philosophical component. Some people find benefit in the massage or meditation or dietary regimes of an alternative practice, but the spiritual or philosophical component does not feel authentic or meaningful to them. They find themselves in a quandary because they want to participate in the helpful aspects, but are put off by the spiritual aspects. To find yourself in any situation that offends your deepest authentic understandings is not healthy. It's better to try to reproduce the effective practices away from the harmful or disturbing spirituality.

Displacement of conventional medicine. Perhaps the most serious deficit of alternative medicine is the fact that some people cease to see conventional doctors when they turn to alternative medicine. This can put their health in real danger. The interventions of conventional medicine have been tested repeatedly and have been shown to produce certain ranges of results repeatedly. Conventional treatments may not provide everything that you want or even need, but they can give you a realistic baseline and assessment of your current condition.

Openness about alternative treatments with conventional doctors. Studies have shown that many people use alternative treatments or go to alternative practitioners in addition to their conventional doctors. But people often don't tell their doctors what they're doing or, more particularly, what supplements, herbs, or vitamins they're taking. This isn't surprising. Some doctors disparage or discourage the use of any alternative treatments. They do it in such a way that patients feel the doctors think they're total fools for believing such nonsense. Sometimes the alternative regimen has made the patient feel better, but their doctor still tells them that they've been conned, and any effect they think they observe is just a "placebo" effect.

Vitamins, herbs, and supplements can have significant, sometimes harmful interactions with other medicines that you're taking, and you may not be aware of these effects taking place. For your own safety, you need to be able to tell your doctor everything you're taking. You should also be able to tell your doctor what activities are improving your situation.

If you've got a doctor who makes you feel stupid or foolish when you speak of these things, you should consider whether you've got a good doctor. Naturally, if the doctor feels that what you're doing is causing you harm, he or she must tell you. But the doctor should back up these assertions with objective information and studies so that you can see that the criticism is not prejudice but rather a thoughtful argument in your best interest.

Getting the Help You Need

You need to find good medical help if you've got a chronic illness or if you're caring for someone who does. Not only must these professionals be competent, but they must be caring, respectful, and capable of listening to you and believing you. You can use your friends and your illness support group, to help find doctors, but you may also want to consider consulting with a medical social worker when trying to find appropriate doctors. You should pay attention to what enters your medical record because it's permanent and may have serious implications in your future treatments or in applications for disability. Finally, use common sense about any alternative treatments you pursue and always continue with conventional medical practice in addition to any alternative methods.

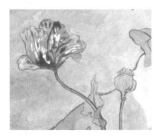

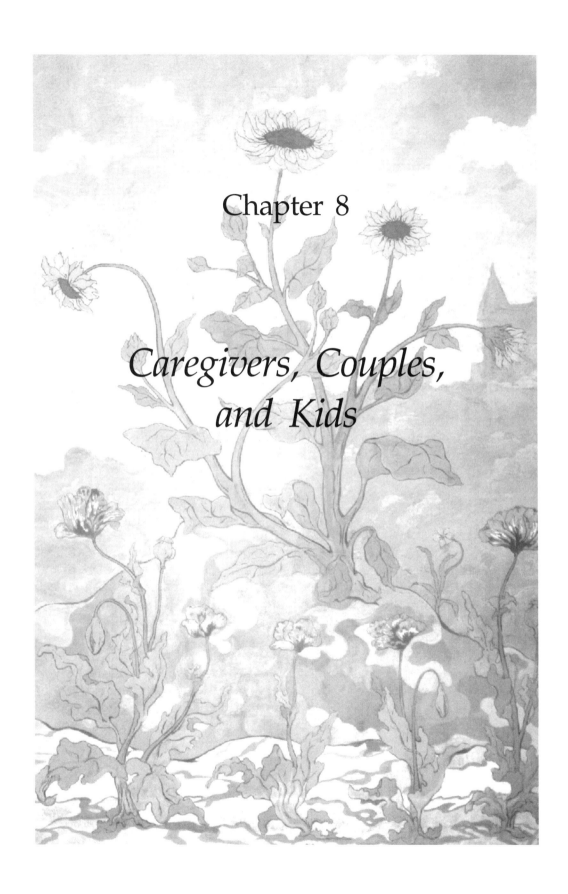

Chapter 8

*Caregivers, Couples,
and Kids*

Throughout most of this book I've been speaking with readers who have a chronic illness. But this chapter is particularly for readers who are caregivers to someone with a chronic illness. Many of the issues of caregiving have come up earlier in the book, but I want to focus on them here from your point of view as caregiver.

Some issues of caregiving are true for everyone. But some issues develop out of the relationship you have with the person who has the chronic illness. The problems and challenges you face are different if you're the spouse of a sick partner, the parent of a sick child, the child of a sick parent, or a friend. First, however, I want to call your attention to things that affect all caregivers.

Issues for All Caregivers

Trauma and Suffering

Vicarious trauma. The people around a person with a chronic illness, most particularly the caregivers, can all experience trauma and suffering just as the person with the illness does. This is called "vicarious trauma." You can suffer trauma because of your intensely sympathetic response to the experience of the person you're caring for, but also because of the many unwanted disruptions and changes that this person's illness may produce in your own life. You suffer pain as you witness the experience of the person you care for, and you suffer pain as your old life is wrenched out of shape or destroyed altogether.

Traumas from the past. Like your care recipient, you've also got your own history of past and present hurts or traumas. Perhaps someone in your family was very sick when you were a child. Perhaps it colored everything about your life then and made you very unhappy or scared. Perhaps it meant that you had to do all sorts of jobs that most of the children your age didn't have to do. These experiences are going to have an impact on how you face the prospect of caring for a sick person now, even though you're no longer a child. Perhaps you were sick yourself as a child, and you've retained strong memories about how lovingly and attentively you were treated. Or on the contrary, perhaps you were ignored or not treated well when you were sick, so you don't have any ideas about how to behave well. This can make you apprehensive that you'll be inadequate to the task, which you know from experience is very difficult yet very important. Perhaps you had a friend or relative in the past who suffered from the same disease as the person you're caring for. Even though there have been many medical advances, you still can't help imagining that your care recipient will experience the disease in the same way. You fear what the future will hold.

Traumas from the present. You may also have traumas occurring right now in the present. Perhaps you're having difficulties keeping your job now. Perhaps you're trying to survive life under a demanding, inconsiderate manager. This can radically affect your attitudes toward having more obligations on the home front. Your life doesn't go on pause just because someone close to you develops a chronic illness. You may have difficulties with arthritis or some other debilitating condition that makes you fear the prospect of new requirements brought on by your caretaking role.

Ignored by others. In addition, while other people may recognize and even sympathize with the suffering of the person you're caring for, not many will think about your traumas and suffering. Because you're known or presumed to care about the sick person, you're expected to fulfill whatever roles are required of you. As a consequence, you may not receive the sympathy, attention, and support that you need.

The necessity of grieving. It's important for you as caregiver to grieve and mourn your losses. Like your care recipient, you can't "go home" again either. Your life has now changed permanently, although not as profoundly as that of the person you're caring for. You may willingly express sympathy for, focus attention on, and help your care recipient, but without proper grieving, resentment and anger can fester. Usually then you feel guilty and ashamed, which eventually makes you even more resentful and angry. Opportunities for misunderstanding and inappropriate behavior multiply. Just like your care recipient, you need to grieve for your losses so you can move forward constructively.

The difficulty of grieving. Grieving can be especially hard for you to engage in, however, because it may seem like a betrayal of the ill person, whom you love and care about. You may feel that grieving for your losses shows that you're being selfish or hostile. You may think that for you to grieve shows that you hold the person you're caring for responsible for your new problems and suffering. It's absolutely essential that you recognize that your care recipient didn't cause anything. It is the illness that has created the difficulties for everyone.

Culturally, it can also be very difficult to grieve. In many social and ethnic groups, if you're related to the ill person, especially if you're a parent or a spouse, you're supposed to sacrifice everything. This is especially true if you are a woman. Moreover, it's supposed to be a willing sacrifice, best demonstrated by not muttering a word of complaint or unhappiness.

Finding a way to grieve. Because it's essential, you've got to find a way to grieve. This needs to be more than a private, internal recognition of your losses in your mind. You need to talk with others about your feelings so that you receive recognition and response. If your family culture makes it hard to grieve openly and publicly, then it's extremely important for you to find other people with whom to talk. Sometimes a family support group for the illness that your family member has can help in this area.

Making use of social workers or family therapists. Social workers or family therapists can also be helpful. These professionals are trained to look at all the systems in the life of a sick person, including those of the family and caregivers. They attempt to create solutions so that all the systems work. They don't just look at a sick person's body, for example, but they also look at how that person manages in the world at large. They understand the effects that illness has on caregivers and the pressures and strains caregivers experience.

Processing the Illness Experience

Developing insight. Like the person with the chronic illness, you need to develop insight into what's happening, what you're thinking about it, and how you're reacting to it. It's quite possible that before the illness, you never gave much conscious thought to your day-to-day life. Now you have to. You need to be consciously focused to carry out your caretaking function, but you've also got to consciously process how you're thinking about the whole experience. Perhaps it's enough to be made aware that you need to do this. But many people need to have some help. Here again a social worker or other counselor may be able to help guide you through the initial steps of developing insight.

Identification and differentiation. Part of developing insight is learning to identify events and feelings and then to differentiate among them. For example, you may find that you become very angry if the person you're caring for remains in bed some days when you think they're perfectly able to be up and around. How do you analyze this angry reaction? You first identify that it's the staying in bed that bothers you. Then you reflect on why you feel this way. Perhaps your mother was sick for a good part of your childhood. You remember that sometimes she would remain in bed for days at a time and that when she did, everything in the household was very difficult. Your father was angry, meals were irregular, your sisters fought. Further reflection allows you to see that you're carrying feelings into the present situation that actually belong to past events. You must try to differentiate the present experience from experiences in your past, seeing that your strong negative feelings come about because of these past events. You need to recognize that the present is a different situation, and you are no longer a relatively helpless child.

Perhaps, on the contrary, your care recipient's remaining in bed makes you feel that you need to stay with them all day. If doing that means that you can't make it to your job, you may begin to worry about missing work so frequently. Here, as you reflect, you can see that the problem is not the fault of the person remaining in bed in and of itself, but whether you can go to work. You're worried about whether the person you're caring for can manage without your being home. The solution to the problem depends on the age of the person and his or her capabilities. You may need outside advice for how best to handle the situation. But the issue ceases to arouse anger simply because the ill person stays in bed on some days.

Realistic Reorganization of Roles

Changing conditions. Even if the individual you're caring for is a small child who required a good deal of attention prior to the illness, the onset of a chronic illness almost assuredly changes the overall amount of work you've got to do. Treatments and care will require time and effort. You will probably have to take your sick child to see doctors, have tests, and so forth. Since you were already leading a full life prior to the illness, this is work on top of work.

Role adjustments. If you're the only other person in the household, you've got to examine your activities and either eliminate some of them or streamline them. In doing this, consider the same issues that are discussed in the activities adjustments of the patient. Try to make sure that you retain activities from all four general categories—activities of daily living, personal enrichment activities, social activities, and work activities.

If you're part of a larger household—one of two parents, for example, with several children besides a sick child—then you need to work with the others in the household to reorganize responsibilities. Often this is a difficult process. It can make a big difference to work with someone like a social worker or a family therapist to identify what jobs need to be done, how often they need to be done, and which members of the household are best suited to doing them under the present conditions. I'll address this issue further below.

Ongoing adjustment process. Because you're dealing with a chronic illness, you'll need to work out a process whereby you can reevaluate and readjust your roles and responsibilities as the person you're caring for experiences changing symptoms. Many chronically ill people go through times of greater functioning when they can participate far more in the affairs of the household. Furthermore it's important for them to do this. But you've also got to be prepared to adapt if your care recipient suffers a relapse or other debilitating emergency. The important thing is not what particular practical arrangements you make, but that you and the others in your household have a way of discussing the situation and redistributing the household tasks.

Specific Caregiving Situations

Using Social Workers or Licensed Family Therapists

In all the situations discussed below, you may find it very helpful to contact a social worker or family therapist. Working through the problems involved with caring for someone you love can be very complex, especially when the care must continue for a long period of time. The issues include both practical and deeply emotional ones as well. These professionals can help you look at all the different systems involved in the care you're providing.

Couples

Change in relationship. One of the most important things that happens to couples with chronic illness is the change in the dynamic of their relationship. Regardless of what existed prior to the illness, you as caregiver usually have to take the initiative, if only temporarily and only in the practical business of life. Nonetheless, this can be an exceedingly difficult change for both you and your partner. Over time, if your affection is strong and you have good communication with each other, this will again change. You and your partner can achieve an egalitarian relationship where all decisions are mutual and each partner contributes equally, though in different ways.

Who's in charge of the illness? When your partner gets sick, you usually have to assume a lot of your partner's responsibilities and tasks. Not only is your partner unable to do these things, but he or she may have also become very unsure and confused. Usually your partner's preoccupied by his or her symptoms and by fear. Your partner may want only to be taken care of. But he or she may also be made very uncomfortable with you taking charge. In the first situation, you may temporarily assume a good deal of direction and control. This may mean that you take over your household and social arrangements, but it may even have to include managing your partner's illness. You may be the one to recommend seeing clinicians. You may be the one who makes sure your partner carries out therapies or takes medication. You may, for a time, seem to do everything. In the second situation, you may need to assume a strong, but very accommodating role. Neither solution is appropriate over the long term. As your partner stabilizes and moves out of the crisis of illness onset, you'll need to consciously return any control of the illness that you've assumed to your partner. Your advice and suggestions may be invaluable, but the person who should make the decisions about treatments and management of the illness itself is the sick person. You want to rebalance your relationship so that it's again between equals.

Who's in charge of your life together? Sometimes illness makes your partner feel dominant. He or she may feel that they have so much suffering that anything they desire goes. This is not appropriate either. While your partner should take charge of the illness, your life together is a mutual thing that requires mutual agreement. You both have to arrive at arrangements for living, and you both have to feel that they are acceptable.

Candid communication. If you've always had a lot of open and frank communication with your partner, then you're much better able to work on all the issues that chronic illness raises. If your relationship has always been more intuitive, based on unexpressed assumptions, and characterized by less open discussion, you've got to begin to transform your style to a more open one. Chronic illness is going to affect so many aspects of your life together that you're going to have to discuss them openly and candidly. Here again you may find that a counselor can help guide you both in methods of talking about matters that are fraught with emotion for both of you.

Roles and responsibilities. Inevitably, you're going to have to readjust your former roles and responsibilities. Your partner may be able to work only part-time or not at all. They may be unable to accomplish most household tasks on a regular, reliable basis. At best, he or she may be able to accomplish only a few, low-exertion ones, such as making the bed or putting away the laundry. The two of you need to talk about what household and work activities have to be done, which can be done less frequently, and which you can perhaps eliminate altogether. You need to discuss objectively, without subtle emotional manipulations, what each can reasonably be expected to do.

This can be extraordinarily difficult work. Everyone has ideas about who they are and what they should be able to do. You've learned gender and relationship roles from the time you were little, and even if you've intellectually rejected many of these concepts, they can still work on you very powerfully. You and your partner are just beginning to grapple with total life changes. For your partner, it's a total identity change as well. Anyone can get angry or depressed when discussing activities that used to be easy, even a pleasure or a joy, that are now impossible. You as caregiver can be appalled by the tasks you apparently have to assume. So it may serve both of you to work with a counselor who can help you address the issues compassionately and objectively.

Setting limits. At the same time that you, as caregiver, must take on many new tasks, you've also got to set limits both internally and externally. When you love your partner, you may want to do everything and be everything for that person. But it's impossible for you to provide the support and care your partner needs plus do all the other tasks that both of you used to do in your life together. Trying to do everything will lead to constant failures, and these will quickly undermine all the good feelings you have.

It's also important for your partner to understand that you've got to set limits. Many sick people initially have to retreat into a sort of self-focused state. They often feel that if their partner really loves them, that person will do everything they need without complaint and without any ill feelings. This is not only impossible, it's not even what either of you really wants. You may be able to work with your partner to recognize that you can only do certain things. But you may need the help of a more objective third party to navigate some of these uncharted waters. Your partner needs to see that you can only be an effective and loving caregiver if you work within your own energy levels and if you have a well-balanced life.

Finances. The illness of your partner almost always means a decline in income and an increase of at least some expenses. Like most people, when a person you love is sick, you probably don't want to think in terms of money or even to talk about money. But money and financial issues can be crucially important. If your partner can't work at all, you need to accept the reality of the situation and start trying to solve the difficulties this presents. Perhaps your partner will be able to work part-time in the future, but for now you need to solve your present budget problems. You need to compare your current income and expenses carefully. Perhaps your partner can get disability. Perhaps you can cut significant areas of expense that are no longer possible or desirable because of the illness. A financial planner may be able to help you assess your current situation objectively and give you helpful management guidance. If you've got little or no income without your partner's salary, you may need to look for employment, even if you've never worked before. A social worker can help you investigate what other options and public aid are available.

Companionability. It's extremely important for you and your partner to find ways to continue to be companions for each other. The illness probably interferes with many of the ways you used to enjoy each other. Perhaps you used to go out to dinner and the movies every week, or you'd go snowshoeing or hiking on weekends. Such activities may be totally out of the question now. But perhaps you can have one night a week when you have a special dinner at home (even takeout from a favorite restaurant) and then watch a video together. Perhaps you can listen to music together or watch a football game and be your own commentators. You can try playing card games or games like Scrabble or Monopoly. Maybe you can read out loud to each other. There are many ways to be intimate together and to talk with each other about things not related to problems or the illness.

Social life. In the past you may have had an extensive social life. Perhaps you and your partner and a group of friends have always enjoyed dinner parties together or other activities. Now your partner's illness makes such get-togethers impossible most of the time. You may be able to meet certain friends at restaurants occasionally, under low-stress conditions. Perhaps you can occasionally have friends in for dessert and coffee instead of an entire dinner. Who your friends are may change after illness because not everyone you know is able to adjust to the illness of your partner. But many old friends want to continue the friendship and will adapt to conditions that work for your partner. In addition, you may find yourself meeting new people who understand about your partner's illness and about what's happened in your life as well. Contact with others suffering the same illness can be very supportive.

It's also important for you to have a social life of your own. Your partner needs to understand that although she or he may not be able to last through a whole evening with friends, you can, and sometimes you need to. You have to be able to go out bowling or have lunch with friends every so often, even though your partner must stay home.

Sexual life. Chronic illness interferes in many different ways with your sexual life. Sometimes your partner is in too much pain or discomfort to even think along those lines. Sometimes fatigue makes it hard to exert oneself sexually. But both of you suffer if your sex life disappears altogether. You need to find ways to be sexual and sensual with each other even if you can't always engage in the same sexual practices and positions you used to. Some couples are very open about sex with each other, while others are more reticent or embarrassed to talk about sex. Some people don't know the many different ways they can bring sexual expression into their lives. This is one of many areas where it may be helpful for you to discuss the issues with a professional, either a social worker or a licensed couples therapist.

Kids

Pain of responsibility. Like most parents, you probably feel responsible for your children and the quality of the life that they lead. When your child gets sick with a chronic illness, you can feel extraordinarily guilty, as though you've failed as a parent. It's easy to believe that the child you love is losing the chance for any life at all.

Worse, your child may be angry and resentful because of the illness and hold you responsible. Children believe that parents create and defend their world. When the world goes to pieces, they can easily feel that the parents have failed. Since the parents also usually feel that they have failed or are responsible, the situation can be very complicated.

You may also suffer from the horrible, sinking feeling that you're never going to be off the hook, that this child will be your responsibility forever. Since this seems like a completely selfish thought and one certainly contrary to the strongly held cultural beliefs of many people, you may feel additional guilt for resenting a life sentence of childcare.

It's enormously important for you to realize that illness is something that happens. It isn't your child's fault, and it isn't your fault. You haven't failed as a parent. It's also important to recognize that the ways you're going to handle the issues related to your sick child are going to allow both you and your child to grow with this illness. Your child is going to get a life by going through the processes outlined earlier in this book. And it can be a full, meaningful life. Moreover, if your child is not severely impaired physically or cognitively, in time he or she will probably need to assume responsibility for management of the illness. If your child is an adult, they may live independently. But even if an adult child continues to live with you, the obligations and responsibilities you have to each other change. You and your adult child will need to work out reasonable household roles and responsibilities the way you would if you were caring for any other adult (see the section below).

Developmental issues. One of the most important issues when you're caring for a sick child is remembering that, even though they're ill, your child is also growing up. All of the developmental issues that occur with healthy children occur with sick children. Sick children, like their healthy counterparts, need to define an independent personality. They need to learn about and explore their universe. They need to create and to play. They must have contact with friends their own age. They undergo puberty and adolescence and are filled with the same moodiness and confusions as their peers, only their feelings are complicated by their illness. They experience sexual maturation and desire.

In every way possible, you want to facilitate sick children becoming adults. It's simply not appropriate to keep them as perpetual children even if they remain in your care into adulthood. This can be very difficult to do, and you may need the guidance of a pediatric social worker, a family therapist, or a child psychologist. Much depends on how mobile your child is, whether your child's able to attend school, and other factors. With the advent of computers, many children have been able to break out of the social isolation imposed on them when they've got to spend a lot of time in bed. Having his or her own phone can also make a big difference in your child's social interaction. You need to think about what materials will enrich your sick child's life, just as you would think about what would enrich a healthy child's life. Your sick daughter may not be able to join a soccer club, but perhaps she can join an online chess club. Your sick son may not be able to play in the school band, but perhaps he can share music he composes on an electronic keyboard via e-mail with his friends.

Handing over illness control. As your child matures, you'll need to involve her or him more and more in illness treatment and management decisions. Eventually your child is probably going to take over control entirely, and you want him or her to be fully familiar with the issues. You want your child to have developed an individual, respectful, friendly relationship with the health-care workers involved in his or her care. By the time your child is eighteen, you should realize and accept as reasonable that your child may make different decisions than those you'd make. This is part of being the independent adult that you want your child to become.

Changing ground rules. As your sick child matures, the ground rules change in areas other than illness. With healthy children, you eventually let them play outside by themselves, cross the road, go visit friends, stay overnight, go to the mall or movies, drive a car. Sick children need to experience the same increases in personal independence. If you find it challenging to extend this kind of freedom to your sick child, you may want to seek some family counseling. Sometimes an objective outsider can help you see how greater freedom will not endanger your child in the ways you fear.

School and other outside activities. If it's possible for your sick child to attend school and participate in activities away from home, this is something to encourage. It allows your child to experience a far more "normal" life, even if she or he is quite restricted at school (must use a wheelchair or carry oxygen, for example). It's true that kids at school can sometimes be very challenging for your sick child, but you still don't want to cocoon your child. If your child is the object of bad behavior on the part of others, you can investigate this and stop it. But many times other children at school will intervene themselves to prevent bad treatment of your child. Many children, at school and elsewhere, are filled with good nature and generosity. They want to include and be friends with your child. If your child seems to have mostly bad experiences, you may want to consult with a pediatric social worker, a family therapist, or a child psychologist on how best to correct the situation. It is also vital to keep school clinicians and other school staff informed and to coordinate with them.

Other children in your family. When you've got other children in your family, it can be very difficult to achieve the "fairness" that everyone desires. Almost inevitably healthy children perceive that caregivers focus more of their time on the sick child. They may be correct. Your sick child may require many trips to the doctor or out for treatment. You may have to spend a good deal of time at home carrying out treatment protocols. And you also have to try to help your sick child make a world to live and grow up in, where much of that world is already supplied for your healthy children.

Here you need to adopt two strategies. First, try to give each of your healthy children regular personal, individual time. This can happen in the conduct of some necessary activity (food shopping, doing laundry, making dinner), but it must involve your focusing on that child and paying attention to that child's interests and concerns. Secondly, you want to involve all your children with each other, including the sick child. Not only do you need the help your children can provide, but your children need to participate in a meaningful way in the life of the family. This includes being involved with each other and with their sick brother or sister. Your healthy children should have things they do with each other and also things that each does with the sick sibling. The sick sibling has to feel that she or he also contributes to family life. Perhaps the sick child can help younger brothers or sisters with homework or read stories out loud to them. Perhaps the expertise the sick child gets with a computer can be shared with older siblings.

Because it can be very difficult to achieve the kind of family interaction and harmony that you seek, you may want to ask help from a family therapist. Such aid can be especially useful if you've got several children passing through adolescence at the same time. Even if you've managed to create strong bonds among them, the stresses felt almost universally by children in our society make this a difficult time for many families. Remember, all children, sick and healthy, have strengths and weaknesses, limitations and restrictions.

Other Family Members

Relationship status. One of the first issues you face when you assume care of another family member is your past status in relation to the sick person. The sick person may have been someone who once had great authority over you, like a parent or a grandparent. The age or generational difference between you and the person you're caring for may make your behavior now seem disrespectful. Even you may regard it that way, and your care recipient is likely to. Or you may actually feel a kind of contempt because this person who once exercised such power in your life is now in need of care. If you felt anger as a child because of a parent's heavy hand, you may feel a kind of revenge in taking over that person's care. A younger family member may arouse parental feelings in you. Being treated like a child may appeal to some people who are sick, especially those in crisis, but it may anger people who don't want to be in a dependent role or feel out of control.

Whatever the age relationship, it's important to remember that your care recipient is an adult, and that you're one, too. Regardless of your prior relationship, you must now act as respectful equals. The illness is not the fault of the sick person, and your decision to provide care should be one you make freely. If you've got serious, unresolved issues with the person who will be in your care, you should work with a professional therapist immediately.

Creating good communications. It's important to begin creating honest, effective communications with the person you're caring for. These will include a realistic acknowledgment of the situation. Since it makes a great difference to start off in the right way, you may want to enlist the aid of a social worker or family therapist to help set up acceptable ways for you and your care recipient to talk to each other.

Roles and responsibilities. You need to discuss with your care recipient what roles and responsibilities each person in the household has. Household roles should not be something taken for granted, for it's highly unlikely you'll all have the same assumptions. In addition, circumstances are likely to change over time. You need to have built up methods and habits of discussing household roles so that you'll be able to make alterations when it's desirable.

Sustainable ground rules. Part of what you'll discuss includes what you'll be able to do and what you can't do. In addition to sustainable ground rules for you, what your care recipient can or will do needs to be clear as well. You both have to assent willingly to these decisions. They won't work if one party accepts because he or she's been browbeaten. Here again an objective professional can sometimes be helpful working out sustainable ground rules.

Assistance. An adult family member receiving your care needs to understand that you may need various kinds of assistance in caregiving. If you're working, you may need to contact the sick person's health-care team about getting assistance. If you can afford to, you may hire people. You may need people to clean the house, prepare meals, or provide company for your sick family member. If it's acceptable to the sick person, you may take him or her to an adult care program away from the home during the day. Whenever possible, try to involve adults you're caring for in decisions related to everyone's living arrangements. They, however, need to contribute to the success of these conversations by participating in a respectful, responsible, equal way.

Your own life. Providing illness care does not mean that the sick person has total call on all your life or time. You must continue at least some of the personal and social activities you used to engage in. While you try to provide your adult care recipients with social connections and pleasures as well, you should be able to enjoy yourself independently of him or her.

Friends

No blood ties. Probably the greatest fear of friends who are cared for by friends is that their caregiver will eventually tire of the job and leave. Friends are not bound by all the cultural imperatives of blood and family. They haven't taken an oath to stick with you "in sickness and in health, until death do you part." Since most people know that even marriage vows often fail under the pressures of chronic illness, what security is there with friends?

Discussion about commitment. As caregiver to a friend, you need to be aware how worry about your commitment can secretly eat away at the confidence of the friend you're caring for. It is therefore extremely important to discuss with your sick friend the level of your commitment and under what conditions that commitment might change. Hard as this conversation may seem, it's essential that both of you know what your commitment is.

Discussion about difficulties. You also need to discuss with your friend the difficulties for you involved with giving care. It's normal for both of you to feel resentful, tired, and bored with each other at times. It's normal for both of you to question the bonds that tie you to the friend you're caring for. You and your friend need to talk about these troubling issues before you can satisfactorily offer them much-needed reassurance.

Reassurance and true friendship. Ultimately you will need to provide a lot of reassurance not only in what you say, but in what you do. Actually, friendship is often stronger and more deeply felt than many family ties. You and your friend have probably built up your friendship over the years, and you share many important beliefs about how you want to behave with each other. Openness in talking about your current situation and matter-of-fact arrangements to deal with practical matters will help reassure your sick friend.

Legal issues. Because you're not related to the friend you're caring for, you may want to investigate certain legal issues with a lawyer. Unless you make specific arrangements, you don't have any formal standing with doctors or hospitals. In cases of emergency, you can't act for your friend, even if you know very well what he or she wants. Such issues can be resolved by health-care proxies and powers of attorney, but you and your friend need to have professional counsel about these matters. It's also wise to involve any close blood relatives of your friend if you're making such arrangements, so that everyone knows what the arrangements are and there are no misunderstandings.

Roles and responsibilities. As with any adult in this situation, you and your friend need to establish your roles and responsibilities. If you've already been living together, you need to adjust what each of you can do now. If you're just coming to live together because of the illness, you need to set up your roles and responsibilities.

Given the fact that you are friends, you may already communicate with each other candidly and authentically. Nonetheless, it can be hard sometimes to be aware of all the issues. A social worker or a family therapist may be able to help both of you identify all the necessary issues you need to consider. Discussions of income and expense can be awkward, especially since your sick friend can probably no longer contribute as significantly as in the past to household maintenance. Disability payments may alleviate some of the shortfall, but the two of you may need to work closely on your budget.

Times together, times apart. It can sometimes be hard to work out how much time you as caregiver should spend with your sick friend. Because of your affection, you may feel that you don't want to do anything without your sick friend. This is not a good idea for many reasons. Having independent friends and activities will help both of you enrich your life together. As the caregiver, these relationships will help keep you from feeling overburdened and your friend from feeling overly dependent. You and your friend both should try to have some life independent of each other. You need to have friends whom you see separately and activities you each engage in on your own. If you're like some people, this is no problem. In the years that you've spent living together in health, you've worked out independent living. Your sick friend's activities and friendships may shift after the illness, but you're both used to leading independent lives. If you've just begun living together because of the illness, this aspect of your joint life may require some attention and work.

Effective, Sustainable Caregiving

As a caregiver you can suffer vicarious and other traumas related to the illness of the person you're caring for. You can also suffer losses. It's crucial that you grieve for both the suffering and the losses. You also need to develop insight about the illness experience as it affects you and your care recipient. Caring for a person inevitably entails changes in what you do. Your roles and responsibilities have to change, and frequently they'll change again in the future. These things are common to caregivers regardless of whom they are caring for. Your relationship to your care recipient creates special issues. Depending on whether you're caring for your partner, your child, an adult family member, or a friend, the issues and challenges you face are different. You'll need to pay close attention to these factors because they'll make a large difference in how you and your care recipient experience your subsequent life together.

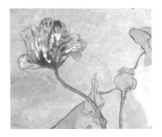

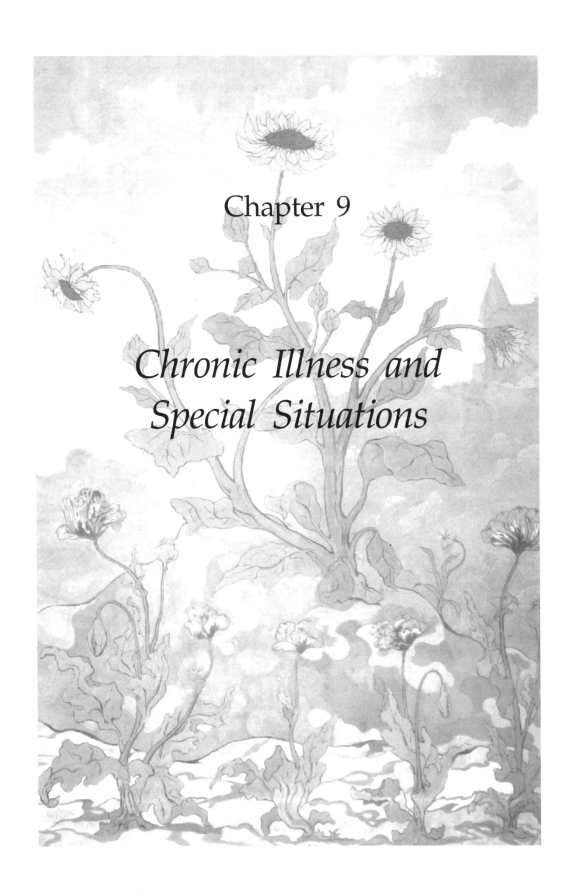

Chapter 9

Chronic Illness and Special Situations

Like everyone else, you're going to have to deal with special situations in your life. A chronic illness can make these more complicated, but you can handle them if you acknowledge that you've got to take extra time and plan carefully whenever possible. Some examples of these situations are:

- **Life transitions.** The major special situations have to do with important life transitions. You decide to get married. You decide to have a child. You move to a new location. You or your partner retires.

- **Illnesses, accidents, surgery.** Certain health-related situations can arise in any life. You get another illness, in addition to your present chronic illness. You have a serious accident. You require surgery.

- **Special environments.** A person with a chronic illness faces certain special problems with environments they live or work in. If you're still working, for example, you must consider your job environment. If you attend college, that's a special living environment.

- **Travel.** Travel puts people with chronic illness under special stresses, regardless of whether the trip is job related, family related, or for pleasure.

- **Weddings, graduations, etc.** There are many special social occasions— ceremonial ones like weddings, graduations, funerals, bar mitzvahs— but also simple ones, like dinner out with friends—that require thought and planning on your part if you're going to survive the event and enjoy yourself.

Two Problems Common to All Special Situations and the Best Solution

Novelty

One of the major stressors that occurs with regard to special situations is novelty. Much of your successful adaptation to your chronic illness comes about when you set up routine living arrangements that fulfill your needs, in the broadest sense, without exhausting your limited energy and capabilities. A special situation falls outside this comfort range. It's not the familiar and habitual, but is new, different, unfamiliar, nonroutine.

Novelty in and of itself can cause anxiety for people who are completely healthy. But it's particularly disconcerting if you've got a chronic illness. This is especially true if your illness causes you to have any kind of cognitive dysfunction, forgetfulness, or confusion. As you face special situations, especially major life changes, you want to think consciously about how the sheer newness of the experience is affecting you.

Unforeseen Stresses

You must also bear in mind that unforeseen, unexpected stresses occur regularly in everyone's life. You can't plan for these stresses except by knowing that they can occur and building some spare, unfilled time into your life. By opening up extra time in your ordinary life, you may be able to absorb these special stresses when they occur. As a person with a chronic illness, you've got less capacity to adapt quickly or sometimes to adapt at all in certain ways. When you're planning for special occasions, try to build in some free time so you have a little wiggle room should an unexpected stress occur.

Planning: the Not-So-Secret Secret of Surviving Special Occasions

Written plans. Planning is your greatest survival tool. As soon as you know that you've got a special situation coming up, you should begin your planning process. I'll go into more detail about specific plans for specific occasions below. What's important in general terms is that you understand how careful, written planning can turn difficult, demanding situations into reasonable and even pleasant experiences.

Go ahead and write out your plans because writing will help you to think about the issues more effectively. It also creates a record of what you need to do, your intended schedule, and a list of actual items—clothes, presents, special equipment, etc.—that you need for the occasion. This record can enable those close to you to quickly learn what you intended to do if you find yourself becoming confused or otherwise cognitively impaired during the course of the event. I'll expand on the role of companions below.

Double your time. However long it used to take you to plan for events before you got sick, double that time. You need a long lead time. Partly this is because you need to make much more precise plans than you did in the past. But partly it's because you're probably not working with the same speed and energy as you used to.

Having enough time to make proper plans will help to calm your anxieties, especially about the issues associated with novelty. By spending time on planning, you'll find that you can actually do more things than you thought you could. In addition, the long lead time allows you to build up energy for the occasion itself.

Activities budgeting. Part of your planning consists of reviewing your regular activities. You need to determine which ones you're going to cut back temporarily so that you can build up energy for the special occasion. Some of you may need to begin building this energy bank account about two weeks ahead of time. Remember, you're not simply putting these activities off until right after the occasion. You've got to eliminate them (temporarily) altogether.

After the event, you're also going to need to keep your activities at a reduced level until you've recovered. You certainly don't want to build up a backlog of obligations that you've simply put off.

It's important to keep your current baseline constitution in mind as you plan, and to balance the four activities groups as you cut back. You don't just eliminate all activities of personal fulfillment or most social activities. You cut back some in those areas, but in work and ADLs as well.

Do You Have a Choice?

The first thing to consider about a special situation is whether you have a choice about participating. Obviously you don't have any choice in whether you have an accident or get sick. And you don't have much choice about such things as moving or retirement. But for many special situations, you can actively decide whether or not to participate.

Benefits and drawbacks. When you have choice, try to think consciously about the benefits and costs for you of participating, and the drawbacks of declining. It's a good idea to write your thoughts down as a way to clarify the issues and focus your thinking.

Major situations. With major life changes like getting married or having children, you want to think very realistically about what you're capable of doing now and what demands your new life would place on you. Since these changes are intended to be forever, you want to know that both you and your partner understand your health situation very well. Prior to making the change, you want to try to work out arrangements for living and managing afterwards. Sometimes an occupational therapist or a social worker can provide important help. These professionals can draw attention to issues that you and your partner may not have considered, and they may be able to suggest potential solutions that you haven't thought of.

Lesser occasions. You'll also want to think about the costs and benefits for lesser occasions. Sometimes an event like a wedding or a graduation is one that you truly want to attend. But sometimes you plan to attend only because other people expect you to, and you're afraid that they will give you grief if you don't. Most of the time, you're probably stuck somewhere in the middle. You would like to attend, especially since it would strengthen your relationships with those involved, but you're worried about how much the event will take out of you.

It's really important for you to weigh carefully the costs and benefits to you of participating. You need to review your activity charts carefully. If you decide to participate, you're going to have to cut down on things beforehand to "save up" for the occasion. Can you do this? And even if you build up energy beforehand, you may find that you're far more exhausted afterwards than you expected. Can you accept that possibility and deal with the recovery time?

Utilize your activities monitor. On just about all occasions, major and minor, you should involve the person you've chosen as your activities monitor. You need to have someone besides yourself assessing the energy the special occasion will cost you. You need to have your monitor help you cut down on your regular activities both before and after the special occasion.

Straightforward communication of your decision. It's possible for you to say no to occasions that you would have gone to in the past. But it's important for you to be clear with the people who invited you that it's your health that makes it impossible for you to attend. You should say how much you'd really like to be with them on the important occasion. And of course you send presents or cards if you can, and make whatever additional gestures are appropriate. After that, if those organizing the occasion don't accept your legitimate and appropriate reasons for not attending, their negative reactions are truly their problem, not yours. This up-front communication is often much easier to say than to do. It takes practice—sometimes months or even years of practice—to learn how to be straightforward about not attending special occasions. At first you're going to feel awkward, embarrassed, and maybe even ashamed. Sometimes it helps to practice in private before you speak to the person whose invitation you're turning down. But you *will* get better at it, especially when you think that it truly is a matter of your health.

Life Transitions

Life transitions are such major events that this book can't examine them in detail. Here are some of the important factors you should consider, however. Try to talk candidly and completely with the people close to you who are involved in these life changes. You should bring to the conversation relevant details about your condition and how you have arranged your life up to this point. The discussions should encompass in fairly precise detail how you and your significant others are going to handle life activities in the new situation.

Marriage

Physical and financial considerations. You and your future spouse need to have a clear understanding of your physical condition now and the prospects for the future. You need to discuss how you'll divide household jobs and responsibilities. You should also talk about how you'll manage financially. If you're working now, the number of hours you work may change in the near future. You and your future spouse should be prepared for the possibility that eventually you may not be able to work at all.

Children and activities. You need to discuss expectations you each have about children, about relations with your families, and about social and activity life. This is extremely important because your energy levels won't permit you to do as much as your future spouse may believe.

Special practical arrangements. You may need to bring up topics such as whether you'll share a bed or not or how often. Many chronically ill people have such disturbed sleep patterns that they really need to sleep by themselves. Sexual matters should be discussed. Food requirements may be an issue. Consider what special needs you have and discuss them openly with your partner.

Do not pass for normal. Candid, complete discussions are essential. If you've got a chronic illness, you must not try to "pass" for normal now with the hope that later you can work things out if necessary. Now is the necessary time. Both you and your future spouse need to plan for reality, not fantasy.

Worth the difficulty. Having this kind of frank discussion with someone you want to marry may really scare you. It's easy to be terrified that the person you love will be completely put off by your situation and leave you. Your fears are normal and very easy to understand. But this conversation is so important for your entire future life together that you must try to have it anyway. It's possible that this conversation may end the relationship, but it will be better for you in the long run to end it now. Moreover, the conversation probably won't be as painful as you fear. Usually the person you love knows that you have a chronic illness, and they love you anyway. In all likelihood this person wants to marry you as much as you want to marry him or her. Your conversation is a matter of working out important details so that they won't come as a surprise later.

Having a Child

Pregnancy or adoption. Contemplating a child involves immediate and long-term issues. Will your chronic illness permit you to sustain a pregnancy? What effect will pregnancy have on your chronic illness? Obviously these are considerations you should discuss at length with your health-care team. If you're contemplating adoption, are you and your spouse viable candidates? Are you willing to adopt a child of another culture, a child with disabilities, or an older child?

Emotional issues. Will you and your spouse be able to sustain the additional emotional complexity that children bring to a marriage? You and your partner each need to think honestly about what will happen if something bad happens to either of you. Suppose you divorce? What if one of you dies? Will you, in your illness, be able to handle a child on your own? Would your partner want the responsibility of a child without your being there to help parent?

Additional activities. You need to think in detail about what parenting means to you in terms of actual activities and behavior. What activities can you do on your own and for what activities will you have to arrange additional assistance? You need to think about how you're going to involve your family and friends. Who of them will be able to help you? Doing what? When? You will not be able to raise a child completely on your own. You need to talk frankly with your activities monitor. Does this person think that you can handle parenting? Does your activities monitor think that you've made sufficient arrangements for necessary help?

Financial considerations. Can you afford to have a child, particularly since you may not be able to work now or possibly in the future? Difficult as it is, you need to think about the possibility that you may not survive until the child reaches adulthood. What will happen to your child if you die?

Moving

Disruption. Nowadays, we tend to treat moving very casually. It's hard to remember that for eons most people lived their entire lives in the same place, rarely venturing farther than a few miles from where they were born. We tend to forget that moving is very disruptive in several different ways. If you move a distance, you've got all the emotional stress of leaving a known community and old friends. But even a move within the same community disrupts your routine life in a major way and sometimes for a significant period of time. This can have a negative effect on anyone, but it's especially difficult for people with chronic illnesses. It's even more distressing if your illness includes cognitive dysfunction, confusion, and forgetfulness.

Is this the best time? If you've got any choice about moving, consider whether you're choosing the right time to move. Moving will deeply affect the quality of your life for a considerable time. Should you move now, or should you wait until you're in a more stable state? Because your symptoms change over time, you may arrive at a time when you'd be better able to handle the stress. On the other hand, you may be at a plateau of symptoms now which makes you as capable as you're likely to be of being able to carry out a move.

Extra work. No matter how much you may look forward to living in a new house or apartment, moving entails a lot of extra work. Most people regard moving as a hateful chore, even if it does give you the opportunity to get rid of unwanted junk. When you have low energy levels to begin with, all the decision making can be almost as draining as the physical tasks you need to carry out. Once you get to the new place, you've got all those boxes to unpack. It's not a bad idea for many chronically ill people to simply plan for taking a year to get entirely unpacked. You may want to consult with your activities monitor during your planning process because you're going to need to save up energy prior to the move and you're going to have to make some long-term energy expenditure tradeoffs during the period of time you're settling into your new place.

Revising your routine and finding your way around. When you move to a new location, you must reinvent your entire activity routine. You've got to develop a new medical team, which can be very difficult emotionally. If you're working, you have to adapt to new job surroundings, a new set of colleagues and superiors, and sometimes a new set of activities as well. You've got to find new local friends. You've got to find out where to shop, do your laundry, fix your car. You've got to learn how to get around. The novelty issue has a great impact here, especially if your illness involves cognitive dysfunction, disorientation, or confusion.

Stocking the new place. Your new dwelling may come with everything you need, but more likely, you'll have to buy appliances, curtains, rugs, furniture, and so on. In other words, you've got an extra set of demanding activities in addition to the move itself and adjusting to the new location.

Planning and information gathering. You want to plan as far in advance of your actual move as possible. Create a folder of information about the new location. Into the folder you'll put lists of things you need to do, items you need to buy, maps, bus or train schedules, etc. Get a copy of the local phone book with the Yellow Pages.

Before leaving your old home, get your health-care team to recommend clinicians in the new location, if they can. Find out where the hospitals are. Inquire whether there's a local support group for your illness. If you can, spend some time in the new location before you move there. Get a map, look around, locate stores near where you'll live. Try driving between your future home and workplace, or practice taking the bus, train, or subway from your home to work.

When you look at your new apartment or house, write down what you'll need to buy in addition to the things you already have. Take measurements to see whether you can use old curtains and rugs, at least temporarily. Try to prioritize your list of necessary purchases so that you're not overwhelmed with shopping and expenses when you're also dealing with the emotional and physical stress of the move itself.

Write everything down and keep all your information in one place.

Retirement

Financial considerations. If you or your partner is retiring, make sure to go over all the implications of this change. Will you be able to manage financially? If your partner is retiring, and you've got a chronic illness, what does this mean in terms of your employment? If you're working, will you have to continue or perhaps even increase the amount of time you spend working? If you haven't been working, will you need to consider doing so? What will the retirement mean for your health insurance? Will you be able to continue living where you do at present, or will you need to prepare to deal with the issues of moving as well as those of retirement?

Emotional considerations. Will retirement change the dynamics of your relationship? If your partner has always been at work all day and you've been at home, will you be able to create new roles and activities when he or she's at home all day? Retirement can be a difficult transition even for healthy individuals. Its emotional adjustments can be especially distressing for those who are chronically ill. Many chronically ill people have been at home much of the time and they often come to regard the home, at least during the day, as their own private place. It can be very disturbing to have your partner, no matter how beloved, in your private space all the time. You and your partner have to work out ways to be together and apart so that your relationship remains strong and supportive for both of you.

Illness, Accidents, Surgery

Another Illness

When you've got a chronic illness, you can easily come to feel that you've had your share of misery, thank you, and that's all the sickness you can or should experience. But the long lives Americans live today mean that it's not unusual for you to contract other illnesses as well. Your new illness will have its own symptoms, but it may also profoundly affect your old chronic illness.

Revisiting the phase activities. You depend on your health-care team to help you deal with all the medical implications of the new illness and its interaction with your other condition. But you've also got to help yourself deal with the emotional and social issues that the new illness brings. Depending on its severity, a new illness can throw you back into some level of crisis. So you need to reactivate the phase activities, starting with phase one. Go back to the bunker and regroup, just as you did with your present chronic illness. Narrow your horizons as much as possible so that you can begin to establish control over your experiences again. As you begin to stabilize, reexamine your activities in light of your new illness. Remember to allow yourself to suffer and grieve for what's happening to you. Work again with those close to you concerning the issues of your life together. In other words, go ahead and work through the phase process again so that you can integrate your new illness into a whole life. Your past experience should help you to do this with reasonable speed, and it should also give you the faith that doing these activities will actually work.

Accidents

Accidents and relapses. The trauma of accidents, particularly serious ones, can increase the symptoms of your chronic illness or even cause a relapse. This is important for you to know because it can sometimes seem like you've been hit by two totally unrelated events—the accident itself and the relapse.

Medical information card. Since you never know when or where accidents will happen, it's important for you to carry on your person essential information that would be vital for a rescue crew, EMT, or hospital emergency room personnel to know. You should carry a card with the name of your illness, primary physician, any special prohibitions for drugs, and other pertinent information.

Prolonged recovery period. Recovery from the physical traumas of an accident can take longer than it would for a healthy person. But what is usually more significant is the emotional stress that accidents cause. Sometimes an accident can also stimulate significant cognitive difficulties, even if such difficulties weren't a great problem in your chronic illness prior to the accident.

Reengage the phase process. Just as when you contract another illness in addition to your original chronic illness, reengaging the phase process will help you cope with a serious accident. You may also find it helpful to see a counselor to help you work through the combined traumas of your accident and its effect on your illness.

Surgery

Effects on chronic symptoms. Surgery can be almost like an accident that you plan. No matter how necessary and how successfully performed, sometimes surgery can cause trauma to your body that can make your chronic symptoms worse. As a consequence, you want to think carefully about any elective surgery. Obviously, some surgeries are absolutely necessary for your overall health, but even those you should enter into with thoughtful, careful planning.

Special arrangements. You very likely will need to make special arrangements prior to, during, and following surgery to meet the needs of your chronic illness. Prior to surgery, you should have a full discussion with your surgeon and anesthesiologist about your chronic illness and the effects that sedation and surgery will have on it. You need to make it clear what medications you can't take and what additional help you may need while you're recovering in the hospital. For example, if you have Sjogren's syndrome, you should make clear your need for eye drops and mouth/throat moisture. The surgeon and anesthesiologist should attempt to find alternatives to typical medications that dry out tissue.

Written notes and companion. Because preparation for surgery is always a stressful time, it's important to write down all the concerns you have and share these with a trusted companion. That companion should accompany you to your discussions with the surgeon and anesthesiologist to keep notes for you and to remind you of issues that concern you. Your companion should be with you as soon after surgery as possible, preferably during recovery. This person acts as your spokesperson and advocate. Many times doctors will note your special needs, but these notes often get lost in the shuffle during your subsequent care. Your companion, who knows your needs, can either inform staff of these needs or contact doctors who can issue the appropriate orders.

Special Environments

Work

Selective disclosure. Most people with chronic illnesses are "out" about their condition to only a select number of people at work. It's my opinion that you should tell co-workers and supervisors about your condition on a "need to know" basis only. When you tell the world, you tend to become a "poster child" for your condition. This characterization can lead to unnecessary stigmatization and misunderstanding for you, and it can be even more oppressive because as poster child, you're often expected to educate people about your illness, advocate for it, and be a model member of those who have it. This can be almost as tiresome as being stigmatized.

Suitable accommodations. It's very important for you to have appropriate working conditions, and many of these are guaranteed by law under the Americans with Disabilities Act. Many employers have to make reasonable environmental alterations to fit your needs. Sometimes lighting needs to be adjusted. You may need changes in workstation organization. You may require a telephone headset rather than a standard receiver model. You may require an ergonomic keyboard. A physical or occupational therapist can examine your work environment to recommend the arrangements most conducive to your health. You may also require one or two short rest periods during your workday. You may require wheelchair access and suitable parking arrangements.

Importance of proper workplace environment. Even if you work only part-time, you spend a good deal of your waking hours in the workplace. As a consequence, it's just as important for you to have appropriate surroundings at work as it is for you to have them at home.

College

Regular and adult students. If you've got a chronic illness and are entering college at the age of eighteen, you're probably intending to live in a dormitory, eat the college food, and live as close to a normal college life as you can. If, on the other hand, you're an adult who is entering college later in life or are returning to college, your situation is somewhat different. You'll probably make your own living and eating arrangements.

Housing. If you're planning to live in the dorms you need to investigate several things in advance to make the experience work. Make sure that your special needs are going to be met. You need to know that your room is suitable. If you're going to have a roommate, the college must match you with a person who will not stay up all night, play loud music, smoke, and so forth. You need to know how to change your rooming arrangement immediately if it proves unsatisfactory.

Food. If you have special food requirements, make efforts to find out ahead of time how the college will meet your needs. Also find out which people you see if things are not working out as promised.

Visiting the college. Most students visit colleges they think they may attend. A visit is a good time to look closely at the dormitory arrangements and at what food will be available. During your campus tours, see the greatest possible variety of living arrangements. Talk with students and the food-service people about the menus available. Ask at interviews with admissions people about the living issues that concern you and how you would be able to change them if you were dissatisfied.

Special study or test-taking arrangements. If your condition requires special equipment for attending lectures, study, or taking tests, you need to determine what the college policy is and what you can do to fulfill your needs. For example, if you have difficulty hearing and need someone to sign for you in class, you must arrange for this with the college administration and with your instructors ahead of time. If you must take examinations on a computer, this also needs to be established ahead of time. If you need longer periods of time to take tests, you must make arrangements with the authorities and with the individual instructors to ensure that extra time.

Even when you have made proper arrangements with the college administration, you should always speak with your individual course instructors before classes start or on the first day of class to make sure they're aware of your special needs. Checking in this way gives you time to straighten out any confusion about rules and regulations before you're actually in a test-taking situation.

Travel

Planning Is the Key

Whether you're traveling for work, family affairs, or pleasure, you've got to plan very carefully if you have a chronic illness. Planning is absolutely key. You can nip potential problems in the bud by mapping out the entire process of your trip and writing down all the particulars in a small notebook that you'll carry with you. If you're traveling with a companion, that person should know to take the notebook and follow the plan if you begin to have cognitive difficulties in the stress of the situation. If you're traveling by yourself, you can use the notebook to orient and calm yourself. With the notebook, you don't need to remember each item every step of the way. You're also going to go prepared for flight cancellations, delays, unforeseen overnight stays, and plans that go awry at your destination.

Mapping your trip. To begin with, draw a map showing where you are and where you're going. On this map, write down how you plan to accomplish every leg of the journey from your home to your destination and back again. This means that you not only make train or plane reservations, but that you also write down how you're going to get from your home to the right gate at the airport and how you're going to get from the plane through the airport to the hotel at your destination. You write down the same detailed information for the trip home.

There may be more than one major step involved in your trip. You may not be flying directly to your destination. You may have to change planes, which means that you must write down how you're going to get from one flight to the other. If you're traveling by train, you may have to change stations before continuing. In that case, you'll need to map out how you get from one station to the other.

Arranging for wheelchairs or electric carts. Your illness may make it highly desirable for you to arrange for a wheelchair or an electric cart at the airport so that you can be taken directly to your boarding gate. If you have to change planes, you'll need to reserve a wheelchair at the next airport so that you can be quickly and safely delivered to your next flight. Not only will you not have to walk long distances, but you'll be able to sit while waiting for your flight to be called. People using wheelchairs are also permitted to board first.

Accommodations. You need to make hotel reservations for the period of your stay. When you do this, make sure to get the name and phone number of the hotel concierge. If you have special requirements for your room or need any other special services, speak directly with the concierge about these matters. You need to be clear about the level of service that's available. Are there restaurants in the hotel, and how long are they open? Is there twenty-four-hour room service? Are bellhops available to carry luggage? What restaurants are near the hotel? You should gather this information when you make your reservations.

The notebook. When you have figured out all of your travel arrangements, write your flight or train numbers and times in a notebook. Note how you're getting from home to the airport, from the airport entrance to the flight gate. Include information about how you get from your flight to whatever transportation you're taking to your hotel. Make sure to note your hotel reservation number, the name and phone number of the hotel concierge, and the names and numbers of any businesses or friends you're planning to see at your destination. And of course, write down everything for the return journey as well.

Your emergency card. In addition to your travel notebook, it's vital that you create an emergency card to put in your pocket, your small purse, or hip pack. This card should have emergency health information on it, plus the most important phone numbers for your destination and those of the people back at home. You can make your emergency card by simply writing down the information on a three-by-five card, trimming the card if you'd like it to be smaller. When you can't find the notebook, it's always good to know that you've got that card!

The contingency plan. You want to be prepared for things to go wrong. Your flight may be canceled. Bad weather may delay you. You may need to spend considerable time in the airport. You may even have go to a hotel while waiting for a substitute flight. Since you're at the mercy of the airlines to make new flight plans, your most important contribution to dealing with unforeseen contingencies are the special supplies you carry. See the section below called "Twenty-four-hour supplies."

Packing. Pack as little as you possibly can. You should take no more than one rolling suitcase to check through on your flight and one small carry-on bag. In addition, you should wear a zipped hip pack or a small, zipped purse with a long strap that you can hang around your neck and down in front of your body.

Try to pack the most comfortable, trouble-free clothing you can find. Knit garments or other materials that require no ironing are ideal. Black or other dark colors hide dirt and serve well in most situations. Your carry-on case, which you've got with you at all times, should have your toiletries, a change of underwear, and whatever you need to get through the night. This last item may be special sleep clothes or perhaps a tape player with a couple of soothing tapes. It's different for each person, but usually there's something that really makes a difference when you're trying to get some sleep.

What you wear. Nowadays most people travel in comfortable rather than fashionable clothing. You can do the same. Dress in several layers so that you can adjust easily to temperature changes. Sweaters or jackets that you can tie by the sleeves around your waist are particularly convenient.

Make sure that you're not wearing anything tight or binding. Wear soft cloth if possible, especially next to your skin. You should wear clothes you'd be comfortable sleeping in, because you may have to do just that. Wear socks that can serve as slippers in case you get bumped off a flight and sent to a strange hotel mid-journey. Wear flat, comfortable shoes that you've long since broken in or soft running shoes.

Twenty-four-hour supplies. Besides your small carry-on bag, you should have a hip pack or small purse. In this you carry your identification, ATM debit card, credit card, necessary medications, and a pack of about twenty $1 bills. You will use these easily accessible bills for tipping. Throughout your trip you'll be tipping cab drivers, porters who carry and check your bags, bellhops, etc., so you'll need a quantity of small bills that you can easily reach. You don't want to have to undo a wallet and hunt around for a bill of the right denomination. You should also have a small envelope filled with quarters for phones and vending machines. I recommend that any person with a chronic illness travel with a cell phone, but you'll need some change as well.

Water. In your carry-on bag or possibly a separate, small handbag you can carry bottled water and food that you can safely eat. Having sufficient safe water is essential. It's enormously important when you are traveling to remain hydrated. You may be able to find bottled water or pure juice to purchase in the airport or train station so that you can stretch out the supplies that you've brought with you. But you can't count on such items being available or your having the time to purchase them if they are. Once you're traveling, your sources of reliable supplies may disappear until you reach your destination.

Food. You should carry enough food that you know you can eat to last you for twenty-four hours. If, in the airport, you find items like bananas for sale, you may want to supplement your stash of prepared food so that you can stretch it further. But you don't ever want to be dependent on what's theoretically available on the plane or train or what's available in the airport or train station. If a connecting flight is canceled and you've got to stay in a strange city, you may also need this food to carry you through until restaurants open at the hotel.

Traveling for work. If you're making a business trip, you should try to arrive at least a day in advance of your business meetings or conference. You'll appreciate having the time to recover from the stresses of the trip. You'll also be much more effective at conducting your business.

Keeping private space. Try not to travel with business colleagues unless they're fully aware of your illness and are willing to accommodate your special needs. Even in that instance, however, try not to share hotel rooms with business colleagues. If you have your own room, you don't have to explain particular bathroom or sleeping habits. Many chronically ill people suffer urinary urgency, particularly at night under conditions of stress. Explaining why you need the bed next to the bathroom and why you go to the toilet five times before going to sleep can be enormously awkward, even if your business colleagues are aware of your illness.

Traveling for pleasure. If your trip is for pleasure, allow time to recover when you arrive at your destination. You don't want to plan any events for the day after you arrive. Besides needing to rest, this arrangement will give you a day in which to think about what you really want to do.

When you're making plans, you should have alternatives in the back of your mind. Sometimes the activities you think you'll enjoy prove to be too much or too jammed together or suddenly unavailable. If you have alternative activities for those times, you won't feel like you've just blown your entire vacation when you're not able to do something special that you hoped to do.

Traveling with a Companion

There's a great deal to be said for traveling with a healthy companion. It can be very reassuring to know that someone's there who can help you out if you get into difficulty and who can make arrangements if you feel like your brain is fried.

You seem normal. Traveling with a companion can be something of a trade off, however. By and large, it's probably not helpful to travel with a person who doesn't know you well. Even if your companion knows you, he or she may not know what you're like under stress. Your friends are used to seeing how you look and behave on your home turf, following your regular routine. There you've got things pretty much under control. In fact, your friends have probably come to think of you as pretty normal. How you look when you're exhausted and what happens when you're stressed and need special arrangements can come as quite a shock. Even if you've tried to prepare your companion ahead of time, he or she may be appalled by how wan and drained you look, how confused you are, or how completely exhausted you can get. You're familiar with these effects because you've experienced them before, but your companion has probably never witnessed you in this state.

Issues of control. This revelation can lead to awkward issues of control. If your companion sees you struggling in a way that's completely unfamiliar, he or she may be liable, out of anxiety for your well-being, to try to assume total control. Your companion may want to run things so that you'll not have to worry about anything. But that may not be at all what you want or need. So it's very important to set boundaries ahead of time. Let your companion know the limits of what he or she should do unless you specifically ask for additional aid.

Fear and flight. Your companion may also react with fear at the responsibility they've assumed. When things get tougher than they've experienced in the past, your companion may want to do nothing more than flee, or at least stay as far away from you as possible. This is why it's very important to know your companion well in advance and to have very frank conversations ahead of time about what they can expect and how you'd prefer they react.

Checking in periodically. It's also important to check in with each other a couple of times over the course of the trip to see how everything is going. Your companion may not be able to read how you're feeling, even though you think it's perfectly obvious. And it's good to keep up on how your companion is doing. For instance, you may not know that your companion doesn't feel free to do things if you can't participate, when in reality you're perfectly happy to have them go off on their own while you stick with more modest pleasures right at hand.

Ceremonial Events

Highly emotional occasions. Ceremonial occasions frequently arouse deep feelings in those who participate. Joy and exhilaration are wonderful emotions, but even happy emotions can be exhausting, especially for people with chronic illness. It's also not unusual for family tensions to simmer just below the surface of an ostensibly happy occasion. Funerals, wakes, and memorial services are often draining, painful occasions. Any big holiday like Thanksgiving can become burdened with expectations for happiness and how everyone's going to act. As a consequence, you should consider carefully what special ceremonial occasions you want to attend.

Costs and benefits. You need to figure out honestly what you can and what you can't do. You must simply decline invitations that you can't sustain. In some cases you may feel that you've got the energy to attend, but you may not particularly want to spend your energy that way. You may have upcoming events that you do want to attend, or work obligations which will require considerable energy. You have a perfect right to make that decision, and you should feel free to decline the invitation.

Use your activities monitor. In making your decision, it may help you to talk with the person you chose as your activities monitor. This person may be able to help you evaluate the benefits of attending by offering a slightly different perspective. Your activities monitor may also be able to help you judge the costs of attending and to select routine activities that you can relinquish temporarily so that you can build up energy for the special event.

Set basic ground rules. If you're part of a family or community with many such special occasions, you may want to think in advance about how far afield, for example, you'll go to attend an occasion. You may want to begin establishing some parameters with your family or community about what celebrations you'll attend so that you won't have to go over the same ground time and again.

If you're a major participant. If you're a major participant—the father of the bride, for example, or the mother of the graduate—you'll probably want to participate regardless of the effect on your health. It's important to remember, however, that sometimes you must say no, even for an important occasion. Much as the people you love may want you to participate, if your health is seriously compromised, they'll have to accept your decision.

How elaborate an occasion? If you do attend, you should first consider how elaborate an occasion is you're signing up for. How involved and elaborate your role is to be may not be your decision alone, but if your participation is important, your input should also be important. The principals need to consider what you are and are not able to do. You'll then need to work with your family members and your activities monitor to arrive at a reasonable amount of participation on your part. You can't, for example, do as much planning and preparation for a bar mitzvah as you would have done if you were healthy. You must either delegate to other family members or hire a person to help you with arrangements.

Factoring in rest periods. Even if you minimize your role considerably, such occasions are always stressful. As a consequence, you must cut back on your regular activities well before the occasion and plan special rest periods during the last few crucial days. After the ceremony, you must plan a rest period before returning to your ordinary life.

If you're an ordinary participant. If you'll be just one of the guests and you decide that you really want to attend the occasion, you should begin your preparations well ahead of time. Write down everything that the occasion requires of you. For example, you need to select appropriate clothes and plan to have your hair washed, cut, and/or styled. You need to select a gift. You may feel that you have to do things like get your car washed. Whatever is important for you to do should go on your list.

Saving energy. During the planning and preparation time, you should begin putting energy in the bank by cutting back on some of your routine activities. It's also usually a good idea at the time you accept the invitation for you to inform your hosts that you may not be able to stay the entire time because of your health. This way they won't be surprised or hurt if you leave early, and you'll feel free to leave when you need to. At the occasion itself, it's wise for you to sit quietly when you can.

Occasions with Friends

Dinner out. One of the most commonplace occasions that can create difficulties for people with chronic illness is dinner with friends. To a healthy person, dinner out seems like a simple pleasure. But your life is hedged with all sorts of restrictions that your friends don't ever think about. You have only a certain amount of energy. You may not be able last for an entire evening out. You may have to be very careful about what, where, and when you eat. Since you became ill, money may have become an issue. You may no longer be able to go to certain more expensive restaurants that you used to frequent with your friends in the past.

Setting parameters ahead of time. If you decide to go out to eat, you need to set up certain parameters with your friends ahead of time. This includes choosing a restaurant that you can afford where they serve food you can eat. It has to have an environment you'll be able to tolerate (a nonsmoking, quiet place, for example). You need to consider how you'll get there and whether you can park right near the entrance. You need to tell you friends how long you can reasonably expect to stay out. If the person you're eating out with is a new friend, you may have to provide a short course in illness etiquette.

Dinner at a friend's house. If dinner is to be at the home of a friend, make sure that your hosts know what you can and can't eat. Even if you don't drink, it's a common courtesy to bring flowers, a bottle of wine or pseudo-wine, or some other small house gift. The advantage of bringing wine or pseudo-wine is that you can build up a small stock of attractively packaged gift bottles so that you don't have to remember to make a special purchase right before you go out.

Other occasions. Sometimes friends invite you over for dessert, for coffee, or to watch a video or TV program. On any such occasion, make sure your friends understand how long you can reasonably expect to stay. You may have to leave earlier than other people do, but you can let your hosts know that if it's okay with them, you'll stay for as long as you can. You may want to think carefully about occasions that involve extensive physical activity. Much as your friends want you to come, they may feel constrained in their own pleasure if you can't participate. If they're willing to accept that you'll sit at the poolside sipping lemonade while they splash around in the water, that's fine. If you think they're going to be made uncomfortable, or worse, if you think they'll pressure you to do more than you're comfortable with doing, then you should decline the invitation.

Gifts, cards, wrapping paper supplies. If it's hard for you to get out shopping, it's very helpful to collect a small supply of gifts, occasional cards, wrapping paper, and so forth. Many people buy these items through catalogs or from companies on the Internet so they don't even have to leave the house to shop. With a supply on hand, you're prepared to respond to occasions with a present or a note without having to make a special trip out to the store. If a friend's in the hospital, for example, you may not be able to visit, but you have a get-well card right at hand and can send it immediately. You also have small gifts immediately available if you make a visit that requires a house present. Having supplies like this is just another way of reducing keystrokes in your life without diminishing its quality.

Coping with Special Events

Special occasions require unusual expenditures of energy from everyone, but they're more demanding of the chronically ill. Significant occasions occur at major life transitions, such as marriage, having a child, and so forth. Surprise occasions occur when you get sick with another illness, have an accident, or require surgery. Work and college environments can also be demanding, as can the problems associated with travel. In addition, there are the many social occasions that occur in your life. Your first concern with any special occasion where you have a choice is whether or not you'll participate. This is a matter of weighing the benefits against the costs. If you decide to participate, you need to make careful, written plans. You need to allow at least twice the time you used to spend getting ready. And you need to build up a certain energy reserve by reducing regular activities temporarily until you have attended the event and recovered from it.

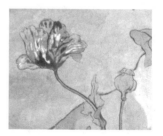

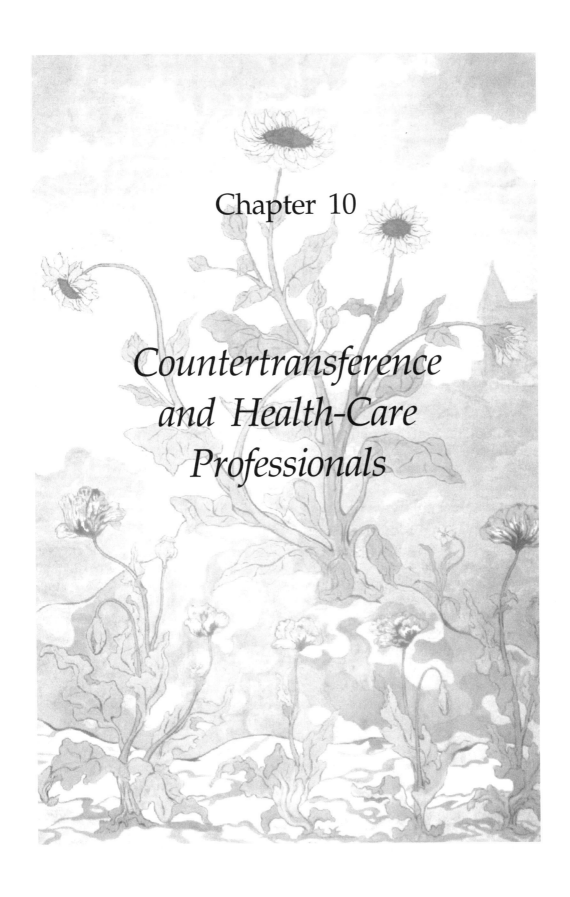

Chapter 10

Countertransference and Health-Care Professionals

You know that you react in some way to everyone you have contact with. Often you have many different reactions, and these change depending on how the other person acts and what the overall situation is. If you go into a store, for example, you will have some reaction to the clerk who waits on you. If the clerk is businesslike and efficient, you probably feel pleased or at least satisfied that the clerk is behaving properly. If you're in a good mood and the clerk smiles and makes pleasantries, you may feel particularly good. It may give you a boost and make you feel even more cheerful than you did before. If you're in a bad mood, you may feel the clerk is irritating and unprofessional. And if the clerk is gossiping with another clerk and makes you wait for attention, you probably feel very annoyed.

You have similar sorts of reactions at home, at work, in your social life—everywhere, in fact. At the same time, although you may pay less attention to it, everyone is reacting to you as well.

This chapter is about countertransference, which deals with how your health-care professionals react to you. You may find that it's helpful to share with your health-care team the information included in this chapter.

What is Countertransference?

Definition. Countertransference is what the health-care profession calls the emotional reactions that clinicians have to their clients. Originally the term was used in psychiatry, and it had a somewhat more narrow meaning. Nowadays the term's used more generally, including all the emotional reactions aroused in any health-care professionals by their clients.

Why is it significant? The reason countertransference has a special name is because health-care clinicians, particularly doctors, used to be taught that as scientific professionals they should not have personal reactions to their patients. They were supposed to suppress or shove aside those few feelings that might slip past their professional guard. The desired response was to regard patients with complete objectivity and determine courses of action on the basis of purely objective assessments. Although this standard has been modified somewhat, the general attitude still prevails.

A problem arises in this strategy because clinicians, as humans, can't just get rid of their personal reactions to others, including patients. When they make the mistake of believing that they have, it's possible for them to act in ways that harm patients. Sometimes they don't even realize that they're acting badly.

Can training teach clinicians objectivity? In their professional education, clinicians learn a great deal of objective information about the human body and mind, about how it acts and what effects different treatments or interventions will have. In addition, because they see many clients in their training and practice, clinicians become accustomed to certain events— copious bleeding, vomiting, seizures, extreme pain, uncontrollable defecation, hysterical behavior, etc.—so that they aren't as terrified or disgusted as most untrained people would be. They often know why these things are happening, which also helps them accept the event. Knowing what's wrong often gives them confidence that they can do something to improve the situation.

So yes, in terms of certain scientific information, clinicians do learn to be objective. And yes, in terms of familiarity with distressing symptoms or behavior, many clinicians are calmer that most lay people would be. But familiarity is not the same as objectivity. It's a habit of mind that comes about because the clinicians are exposed to the situation frequently enough to have personally comfortable rationalizations for it.

Our culture demands objectivity. In addition to their training, doctors and other health-care professionals are told by the culture that they must be objective scientists. We who live in this culture trust doctors to do things to our bodies and minds because we believe that science provides answers. We believe health-care professionals are acting scientifically.

Doctors want to believe this, too, but most know that medicine does not always rely on hard facts. Medical professionals use their judgment, they use their intuition, and they make informed guesses or hypotheses utilizing their professional training. Much of that training, after all, has taught them how to reach reasoned conclusions. Doctors also go on the basis of what they know (or think they know) about a particular patient. They're often right. But in their actions they aren't always operating objectively. They're also making subjective assessments.

To react is to be human. Clinicians are constantly reacting to their patients. It's not some rare thing that happens only occasionally. Indeed, these reactions often help clinicians figure out what's wrong with their patients. They can help clinicians grasp which treatments are working and which aren't and why, even if the patient can't explain in words.

In addition, however, clinicians react to their patients in other ways. They notice when their patients are boring or whiny or repetitive. They may have feelings of disgust or revulsion about some patients. They may be afraid of them. Clinicians can also, of course, be amazed by patients, delighted with them, in awe of them, or admiring of them.

How Does Countertransference Operate?

Problems caused by failure to acknowledge countertransference. When clinicians fail to recognize their countertransferential feelings, they are unable to deal with these emotions in a positive way. Instead, for example, feelings of disgust or disapproval can cause clinicians to pull back from patients, to avoid examining them as closely or as frequently as they would patients who do not produce these reactions. It can blind clinicians to significant information that patients may be trying to convey. In extreme situations, countertransference may make clinicians avoid seeing such patients altogether. They may either refer them to other doctors or dismiss the patients' concerns as being "all in their mind."

Even positive feelings can distract clinicians from hearing or seeing all the information they need to make informed interventions. Admiration for how cheerfully a patient appears to be handling kidney failure, for example, may blind a doctor to subtle indications of growing depression or instances of noncompliance with treatment.

Distraction from patient. Countertransferential issues can distract clinicians from paying attention to their patients. Instead, the clinicians may begin focusing on their own reactions and what they're going to do about them. In essence, they only selectively hear or see the client in front of them.

Disbelief. Some clinicians don't believe what chronic illness patients tell them unless the clinicians can corroborate it at the time of the visit by physical examination or specific test results. Chronic illness patients almost always report symptoms that aren't apparent at the time of the visit, so clinicians who rely wholly on testing and observation will tend to distrust or disbelieve their patients. Such attitudes aren't lost on the patients, who can suffer mild or severe iatrogenic trauma in response. It can also cause patients to begin misreporting in order to please clinicians whom they're afraid of offending.

Intolerance of suffering. On some level, most health-care professionals have entered the field because they want to relieve suffering. The acute illnesses that form the model for Western medicine usually allow clinicians to do very specific things to relieve suffering. If patients survive an acute illness, they usually cease to suffer from that disease. But with chronic illness, suffering is ongoing. Sometimes it even intensifies. Some clinicians can't tolerate this, which means they have a very difficult time tolerating the individuals who continue to suffer despite the clinicians' best efforts. If clinicians are unable to deal with suffering, it makes it even more difficult for patients to learn to work with their suffering. Such patients lack the powerful model that clinicians can provide.

Intolerance of chronicity and ambiguity. Chronic illnesses are by definition chronic—the doctor won't ever achieve a cure. This can be very difficult for clinicians, as a cure is the one sure sign in Western medicine that the doctor has been successful. Everything conspires to make doctors who don't cure patients feel like failures. The patients often feel such doctors have failed. The patients' families can feel the doctors have failed. The culture says the doctors have failed. Small wonder then if doctors feel like failures when they don't achieve a cure. It takes a special kind of clinician not to feel depressed, discouraged, or irritated when patients don't get better.

Chronic diseases are also ambiguous. Not enough is known about them, and their symptoms change all the time. This, too, bothers some clinicians who want a clear linear progression to health in their patients. Ambiguous conditions are frustrating.

Since both the chronicity and ambiguity of their conditions are terrible stumbling blocks for the patients, it's crucially important for clinicians to learn to understand them and deal with them. Not only do clinicians provide physical interventions for patients, but their behavior and attitudes are constant models for patients and those close to the patients.

Avoidance of chronic illness patients. Because chronic illnesses don't fit neatly into the standard acute model of disease in Western medicine, some clinicians may assume that the symptoms are psychological in origin. Some may be so uncomfortable with the chronic experience that they begin to treat chronically ill patients with suspicion, distaste, or even as individuals who are malingering or creating their own physical symptoms.

Some clinicians may also look down on other clinicians who treat such diseases. This lowers the professional status of clinicians who have an interest in chronic illness. Being human, clinicians seek honor and admiration just as others do. Some of these clinicians will tend to avoid working with populations who are believed to have self-inflicted or nonexistent problems.

Countertransference Used Effectively

Countertransference can be a useful tool. Contrary to earlier perceptions that countertransference is always undesirable, it can actually help clinicians do a better job. This benefit does require that clinicians recognize these feelings when they arise and that they process them effectively. Clinicians have to do double work. They must listen attentively to their patients to hear on all levels what the patients have to say. They've also got to "listen" to themselves. Later, when they have time to reflect, they must examine their feelings and develop insight and understanding as to why they're having these feelings with this patient in this situation. On the basis of this insight, they must try to see whether and how they can use what they've learned about themselves to help their patients.

Egalitarian relationships. Acknowledgment and acceptance of countertransference helps to establish the egalitarian relationships that produce the most effective therapeutic situations between clinicians and patients. When some clinicians consistently behave as beings superior to their patients, they set themselves apart in ways that can permit them to behave badly or inconsiderately. They certainly wouldn't want such behavior directed at them, but they believe that they aren't like their patients, so it doesn't matter. It's extremely important for patients and clinicians to recognize that they differ only in expertise. The clinician has acquired a great deal of knowledge and experience that the patient doesn't have, but the patient is rapidly accumulating specific experiences the clinician doesn't have. Regardless of distinctions in knowledge, both patient and clinician are the same in humanity.

Especially when dealing with the long-term problems and adjustments associated with chronic illness, patients and clinicians must become equal partners. They differ in knowledge, but they must be respectful of each other. It is clear, especially with regard to the psychological and social-interactive aspects of chronic illness, that a strong egalitarian relationship between patient and clinician is more effective than any particular variety of therapy the clinician employs.

Typical Countertransferential Issues by Phase

Phase One: Crisis

Emotions. The urgency and desperation of patients in phase one can arouse revulsion, fear, and anger in clinicians. Such feelings occur on a continuum, of course. Some clinicians will only have twinges of fear, for example, while others will be very frightened. Clinicians may share cultural biases against the chronic illness that a patient appears to have. Clinicians may not be able to identify what's wrong and fear that the illness may be something catching. The absence of stable, measurable symptoms may frustrate and anger clinicians. They may interpret a patient's complaints as a form of malingering or social irresponsibility. The degree of suffering in phase one patients can be so intense that clinicians may want to reject or pass them along to other practitioners.

It's possible for the patients' traumas to trigger dormant traumas in the clinicians' lives. "Medical school syndrome" can also come into play, as the clinicians begin to imagine the patients' symptoms in their own bodies.

Actions for clinicians. Clinicians can work through almost all of these emotions by thoughtful examination. Where clinicians are ignorant about an illness—which produces many negative emotions—they should be honest about their lack of knowledge with themselves and with their patients. They should seek out information from others and refer their patients to specialists as necessary. Clinicians should adopt a spirit of humbleness before the complexity of the patient's situation and honor the work they do with the patient. Most of all, they should affirm the reality of the patient's experience and respect the patient's communications, no matter how awkwardly expressed. They should seek to model helpful behavior in their own actions. They should also take seriously their role as witness for their patients' experiences. Acting as a witness of the chronic illness plays a significant part for the patient throughout the phase process. Witnessing makes real what is real but is not always regarded as real. A witness not only sees that something real is happening and how it's happening, but by paying attention to what is happening helps to give the events importance. Witnessing calls attention to things that others often want to hide or ignore.

Actions for patients. When you feel that your clinician has reacted inappropriately, you should say so. You should talk about what bothers you. You've gone to the professional because that person has different, more specific information than you do and exposure to a wider range of illness experiences. But that is no excuse for clinicians' behaving in any way that demeans you. If they will not talk honestly with you, you should think about finding a different clinician. Similarly, if the clinician is helpful, please share this information, too.

Phase Two: Stabilization

Emotions. Clinicians may have many of the emotions typical of phase one, especially if they're seeing the patient for the first time. In addition, they may often find themselves in conflict with patients, with their families, or with their own professional colleagues. Phase two patients have stabilized, but they still have not returned to normal. It is easy for people to consider the clinician a failure. This often includes the clinician, who wanted the interventions and treatments employed so far to achieve a cure or indicate clear movement toward one. Sometimes the healthy seeking behavior of phase two patients, who are urged on by their significant others to get cured, leads them to reject the clinician as inadequate. They terminate the relationship, which can offend and hurt the clinician.

Because they treat phase two or three chronic illness patients, clinicians can suffer vicarious trauma in relation to their profession. The crisis of phase one can appear to be the practice of serious medicine, but the long trek through phase two and three can appear to be useless encouragement of a questionable clientele.

Actions for clinicians. If clinicians have become acquainted with the phases that chronic illness patients experience, they're better equipped to deal with their feelings and to help their patients. They can recognize that much of the conflict stems from the fact that the patient has not and probably won't normalize. This source of conflict will continue until patients and their significant others travel through phase two and arrive at the recognition of chronicity that characterizes phase three.

If patients' seeking behavior is so strong that they break with the clinician, the clinician can let them go without offense. When they understand the phases of chronic illness, clinicians can see the healthy aspects of the patients' search. At the same time they should make it apparent to patients that the door is open for their return should they desire to do so. It can be very reassuring to the patient if the clinician makes a phone call to find out how the patient is doing sometime after the patient has left. Such action may even encourage the patient to return.

Clinicians need to realize what is happening when some of their colleagues treat them with disregard. They need to join with others in similar practice, just as their chronic illness patients need to find others of like kind to support and encourage them.

Actions for patients. You need to recognize that, just as you do, clinicians can become frustrated because there is no cure for your condition. At the same time, this should not lead to withdrawal or growing indifference. Ultimately you've got to come to terms with the chronicity of your condition, but as you're getting to that place, you may want to seek help from a variety of clinicians. If you've had a good and caring clinician and left that person, you should have no problem if you decide to resume treatment with that clinician.

Phase Three: Resolution

Emotions. Clinicians often share the feelings of terror and sadness that phase three patients feel as they recognize deeply that they "can't go home again." Clinicians frequently feel inadequate to the task of helping their patients endure the dark night of the soul. Phase three is frequently a time when clinicians want to withdraw, saying that these emotional and philosophical or spiritual issues aren't their areas of expertise. As a result they can reject their patients because they fear having to examine their own existential issues.

Actions for clinicians. Clearly clinicians need to do some examination of their own issues, including their existential issues. If their patients can do it (and they must), so can the clinicians. They won't arrive at the same answers, but experiencing some of the same journey will make it easier for the patients. Clinicians can gain one handle on this by accepting the task of spending time in the tunnel with the patient. They can project faith, even as they themselves are seeking it.

Actions for patients. It's important for you to know that everyone must eventually face serious existential questions, including your clinicians. You need to realize that your clinician can have the same fears and terrors you do. But your clinicians are in their business because they've got hope and faith that you can work through to a better place and a more complete life.

Phase Four: Integration

Emotions. By phase four, clinicians can feel a mixture of great attachment to their patients, enormous pride in their achievement, yet a sense of loss or grief as they depart.

Actions for clinicians. Phase four is a time for sending the patient forth. It's usually not difficult to overcome feelings of sadness that the patient is leaving because clinicians have pride in the patient's achievement. In addition, many patients have developed such a warm bond that they periodically contact clinicians just to keep in touch. Nonetheless, clinicians need to engage themselves consciously in the departure and resolve any lingering countertransferential issues they may have.

Actions for patients. You should know that your clinicians are proud of you, happy for your achievement, and delighted to see you able to take charge of the new life you've constructed. Your affection will often mean that you'll continue letting clinicians know through occasional e-mails or seasonal cards how things are going.

Clinicians Are Human, Too

Clinicians react emotionally to their patients all the time, just as all human beings react to each other. Traditionally, the medical establishment used to discourage clinicians acknowledging, let alone using, these emotions because clinicians were supposed to be entirely objective and scientific in relation to their patients. Nowadays most professionals recognize that such objectivity doesn't exist. On the contrary, when clinicians don't recognize and process their emotional reactions to patients, they may harm them. They may not treat them in the egalitarian manner that is most effective, especially with chronic illness patients. Clinicians should identify their reactions to patients, process them, and seek to turn their emotional reactions to positive use, if possible.

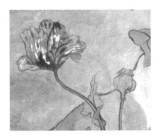

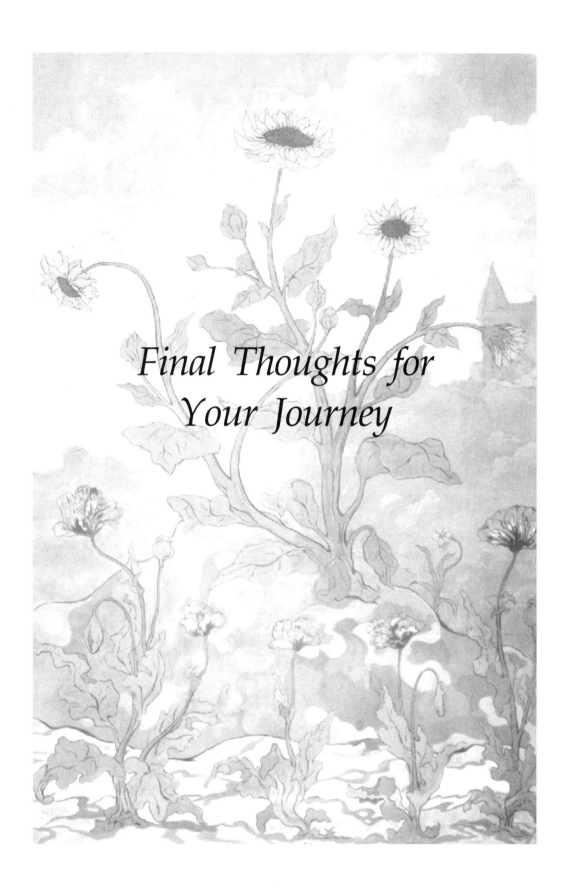

*Final Thoughts for
Your Journey*

The Phase Journey Map

Now that you've read through this book, I suggest that you take a few minutes and review the summary sections of each of the phase chapters. You can think of these summaries as a roadmap for your journey through the phases. Or you can think of them as operating instructions. In this chapter you'll find a breakdown of these summaries, and you might considering copying them and then taping these copies on a wall or putting them on your refrigerator door. This way you can check in easily on where you are, where you've been, and where you're going.

Typically, when people are introduced to the phases, they place themselves further along the phase process than they actually are. That's a very normal, human thing to do. We always want to be further along on any trip. It's a kind of an "are we there yet?" approach. Regardless of where you place yourself in the phase process, it is worth reading or rereading material about the earlier phases. There are many suggestions in those sections that will help you where you are right now and will certainly help you if some unforeseen crisis occurs in your life.

Phase One

Goal: Contain the crisis.

Actions: Put together a reliable, caring health-care team, with a team leader you like and trust.

Follow clinical instructions faithfully and report to your team leader regularly.

Learn about the nature of chronic illnesses and the phases.

Observe and chart your activities, symptoms, feelings and how they are interrelated.

Go into the bunker. Reduce your activities to a level you can sustain. Keep tracking your activities, symptoms, and feelings.

Begin a personal narrative.

Begin establishing new relationships with the other people in your life and workplace.

----➤   **Learn to allow your suffering.**

Phase Two

Goal: Stabilize and begin restructuring your life.

Actions: Commit to a period of "monastic" life.

Reassess your physical situation, your medical treatments, protocols, medications.

Identify your activities by activity group. Make sure your activities are balanced among the four activity groups.

Begin defining boundaries of your new life, including activities from all four activity categories.

Develop your skills of self-observation.

Work to maintain your insights. (This one's difficult to do!)

Start clarifying your values and developing new norms.

Work with significant people in your life regarding the fact that you're not going to return to "normal."

Make time to grieve your losses and suffering.

----▶   **Learn to regard your suffering with compassion.**

Phase Three

Goal: Maintain insight, develop meaning, construct a new self.

Actions: Begin assuming management of physical care coordination, if possible.

Actively grieve for losses and suffering. (This is a tough one.)

Commit to the "time in the tunnel." Explore existential questions and find meaning.

Analyze what exactly you've lost and what you haven't.

Begin constructing a new self, using your developing skills of insight, issue reframing, antithetical experimentation, and creative activity.

Assess everything about your new self and your ideas about meaning for complete personal authenticity.

Assert that you're not a burden to others but simply a person with particular needs.

Find ongoing methods with your significant others to adapt to the changing conditions of your life together.

Rely on supporters and explore reincorporation of old friends or family members.

Consider political action related to your illness.

Stand with your new self without apology.

---▶   **Learn to meet your suffering with respect.**

Phase Four

Goal: Integrate your illness into a whole and meaningful life.

Actions: Accept that you may experience phase four only periodically.

Stay attuned to your illness cycle, maintain regular medical reviews, and keep abreast of developments in your illness.

Monitor your activities to keep within your physical boundaries and to maintain a balance of activity over the four activity categories.

Continue to explore and grow creatively and spiritually.

Maintain your new self and strive for your new "personal best."

Commit to your daily acts of bravery as matters of free will.

Expand your meaning development to encompass the whole world as well as yourself, from the smallest tasks to universal considerations.

Expand your social horizons as much as your condition will permit.

Keep in continuous touch with your family, partner, and friends.

Recruit new supporters and integrate old ones who wish to reconnect to your life.

Engage in social action.

Seek authentically meaningful work.

Commit to living with the paradox and in the mystery.

----▶   **Learn to integrate your suffering into a whole life.**

Respect Yourself, Respect Your Efforts

This journey isn't easy and it's not for the faint of heart. It takes tremendous courage to allow your suffering, to show genuine compassion for yourself, and to respect yourself for what you have endured. As you've learned by now, not everyone in your pre-illness life will make the journey with you. But at the same time, you've met some very important new people—those who are sharing your journey because they're ill too, or people who like you for who you are and therefore want to share your journey.

No matter how you construct or conceive it, faith is essential to your trip. And the most essential pillar of that faith must be your faith in yourself. This faith will grow as you acquire the ability to see and understand your situation, as you learn how to cope with your particular needs and desires, as you discover the authentic person you are now, and as you learn to tolerate the chronic and the ambiguous. Faith doesn't come with flashes of lightning, huge breakthroughs, or amazing epiphanies. If something like that happens to you, enjoy the experience. But the real growth of faith happens like all growth in nature, slowly, over time. Real faith emerges gradually out of your many small, daily acts of courage when you stand with yourself.

If you feel shaky, remember that you're not alone. Sooner or later, all of us will be on this journey just like you are. You already know people on the road who want to support you, just as you want to support them. Everyone needs to borrow the strength and faith of others at times, just as everyone shares faith and support when they're feeling strong and confident. When you're feeling unsure, remember to reorient yourself by looking at your phase roadmap. And remember, we're on the road with you, sharing the journey.

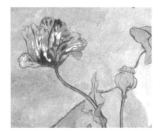

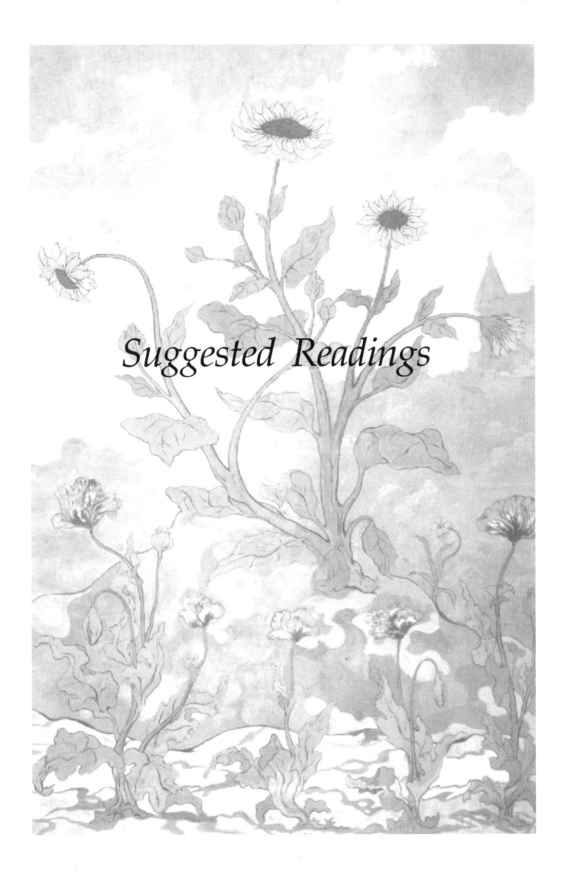

Suggested Readings

Chester, L. 1987. *Lupus Novice*. Barrytown, NY: Station Hill Press, Inc.

Cousins, N. 1979. *Anatomy of an Illness as Perceived by the Patient*. New York: Norton.

Duff, K. 1993. *The Alchemy of Illness*. New York: Crown Publishers, Inc.

Estroff, S. E. 1993. Identity, disability, and schizophrenia: The problem of chronicity. In *Knowledge, Power and Practice,* edited by S. Lindenbaum and M. Lock. Berkeley: University of California Press.

Fennell, P. A. (in press) *Understanding Chronic Syndromes: The Four Phases of Change*. Mahwah, NJ: Erlbaum Publishers.

———. 1993. A systematic, four stage, progressive model for mapping the CFIDS experience. *The CFIDS Chronicle*. Summer, 40–46.

———. 1995. CFIDS, socio-cultural influences and trauma: Clinical considerations. *Journal of Chronic Fatigue Syndrome*. 1:159–173.

———. 1995. The four progressive stages of the CFIDS experience: A coping tool for patients. *Journal of Chronic Fatigue Syndrome*. 1:69–79.

Fennell, P. A., L. A. Jason, and S. M. Klein. 1998. Capturing the different phases of the CFS Illness. *The CFIDS Chronicle*. 11:13–16.

Frankl, V. E. 1959. *Man's Search for Meaning*. Boston: Beacon Press.

Garrett, L. 1994. *The Coming Plague: Newly Emerging Diseases in a World Out of Balance*. New York: Farrar, Strauss and Giroux.

Good, B. J., and M. J. DelVecchio/Good. 1993. Learning medicine. The constructing of medical knowledge at Harvard Medical School. In *Knowledge, Power and Practice,* edited by S. Lindenbaum and M. Lock. Berkeley: University of California Press.

Katz, M. 1997. *On Playing a Poor Hand Well*. New York: W. W. Norton & Company.

King., M. L. Jr. 1986. *A testament of hope: The essential writings and speeches of Martin Luther King, Jr*. New York: Harper Collins.

Kleinman, A. 1980. *Patients and Healers in the Context of Culture*. Berkeley: University of California Press.

———. 1988. *The Illness Narratives*. New York: Basic Books.

Kornfield, J. 1993. *A Path-with-Heart*. New York: Bantam Books.

Kreinheder, A. 1991. *Body and Soul: The Other Side of Illness (Studies in Jungian psychology)*. Toronto, Canada: Inner City Books.

Kubler-Ross, E. 1970. *On Death and Dying*. New York: MacMillan.

Kushner, T. 1993. *Angels in America.* New York: Theater Communications Group.

Lamott, A. 1999. *Traveling Mercies: Some Thoughts on Faith.* New York: Anchor Books.

Levine, S. 1979. *A Gradual Awakening.* NY: Doubleday.

Mairs, N. 1996. *Waist-High in the World: A Life Among the Nondisabled.* Boston: Beacon Press.

Mandela, N. 1994. *A Long Walk to Freedom: The Autobiography of Nelson Mandela.* Boston: Little Brown.

Matsakis, A. 1992. *I Can't Get Over It: A Handbook for Trauma Survivors.* Oakland, CA: New Harbinger Publications, Inc.

Melecki, J. J. 1994. Jungian perspective on suffering and pain in physical illness: A story of Esther. *The Journal of Pastoral Counseling,* Vol. 29:43–71.

Mukand, J. (Ed.). 1994. *Articulations: The Body and Illness in Poetry.* Iowa City: University of Iowa Press.

Nouwen, H. 1979. *The Wounded Healer.* New York: Doubleday Dell Publishing Group.

Pitzele, S. K. 1985. *We Are Not Alone: Learning to Live with Chronic Illness.* New York: Workman.

Register, C. 1987. *The Chronic Illness Experience.* Center City, MN.

Sontag, S. 1977. *Illness as Metaphor.* New York: Farrar, Straus and Giroux.

Wells, S. M. 1998. *A Delicate Balance: Living Successfully with Chronic Illness.* New York: Insight Books.

West, C. 1993. *Race Matters.* Boston: Beacon Press.

Wilson, J. P., and J. D. Lindy. Eds. 1994. *Countertransference in the Treatment of PTSD.* New York: The Guilford Press.

Woolf, V. 1948. "On being ill". In *The Moment and other Essays* edited by L. Woolf. New York: Harcourt Brace Jovanovich.

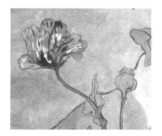

About the Author

Patricia Fennell, MSW, CSW-R, is the President of Albany Health Management Associates Inc., a multitask organization that engages in counseling, health-related research, professional training, community education, and chronic illness retreats. For more than fifteen years Ms. Fennell and her staff have been working to alleviate the suffering created by trauma and chronic illnesses including chronic fatigue syndrome, fibromyalgia, and other chronic syndromes. She is also the Senior Clinical Consultant at the Capitol Region Sleep/Wake Disorders Center, in Albany, NY.

Ms. Fennell, who resides in Albany, N.Y., is an innovator in the chronic illness and mental health fields. She created the internationally recognized Four-Phase Model for understanding and treating chronic syndromes. The model is used by medical and counseling clinicians, medical researchers, and patients in the U.S., Canada, Australia, and Europe. Fennell's academic book on the same subject is currently in press.

Ms. Fennell, a popular speaker, gives numerous presentations and workshops for both professionals and patients. She provides consultation for a variety of organizations, continues to see patients and supervise other clinicians, and, utilizing original content and curriculum, administers a two-year training program in chronicity studies.

Some Other New Harbinger Titles

The Trigger Point Therapy Workbook, Item TPTW $19.95

Fibromyalgia and Chronic Myofascial Pain Syndrome, Item FMS $19.95

Kill the Craving, Item KC $18.95

Rosacea, Item ROSA $13.95

Thinking Pregnant, Item TKPG $13.95

Shy Bladder Syndrome, Item SBDS $13.95

Help for Hairpullers, Item HFHP $13.95

Coping with Chronic Fatigue Syndrome, Item CFS $13.95

The Stop Smoking Workbook, Item SMOK $17.95

Multiple Chemical Sensitivity, Item MCS $16.95

Breaking the Bonds of Irritable Bowel Syndrome, Item IBS $14.95

Parkinson's Disease and the Art of Moving, Item PARK $15.95

The Addiction Workbook, Item AWB $17.95

The Interstitial Cystitis Survival Guide, Item ICS $14.95

Illness and the Art of Creative Self-Expression, Item EXPR $13.95

Don't Leave it to Chance, Item GMBL $13.95

The Chronic Pain Control Workbook, 2nd edition, Item PN2 $18.95

Perimenopause, 2nd edition, Item PER2 $16.95

The Family Recovery Guide, Item FAMG $15.95

Healthy Baby, Toxic World, Item BABY $15.95

I'll Take Care of You, Item CARE $12.95

Call **toll free, 1-800-748-6273,** or log on to our online bookstore at **www.newharbinger.com** to order. Have your Visa or Mastercard number ready. Or send a check for the titles you want to New Harbinger Publications, Inc., 5674 Shattuck Ave., Oakland, CA 94609. Include $4.50 for the first book and 75¢ for each additional book, to cover shipping and handling. (California residents please include appropriate sales tax.) Allow two to five weeks for delivery.

Prices subject to change without notice.